ANGLO-INDIAN CUISINE
A LEGACY OF FLAVOURS FROM THE PAST

AUTHENTIC ANGLO-INDIAN RECIPES

ANGLO-INDIAN CUISINE—A LEGACY OF FLAVOURS FROM THE PAST was selected as the *'WINNER FROM INDIA'* under the Category: *BEST CULINARY HISTORY BOOK* by GOURMAND INTERNATIONAL SPAIN, *GOURMAND WORLD COOK BOOKS AWARDS 2012*

BRIDGET WHITE

authorHOUSE®

AuthorHouse™
1663 Liberty Drive
Bloomington, IN 47403
www.authorhouse.com
Phone: 1-800-839-8640

Bridget Kumar
No. 6 / A, 1st A Main Road,
S T Bed Extn, Opp. Caravel Info Systems,
Koramangala 4Th Block, Bangalore 560034. India.
Phone: +91 80 25504137 / **Mobile:** +91 9845571254,
Email: bridgetkumar@yahoo.com / bidkumar@gmail.com
www.anglo-indianrecipes.blogspot.in
www.anglo-indianfood.blogspot.in

Published by AuthorHouse   12/19/2012

ISBN: 978-1-4772-5163-8 (sc)
ISBN: 978-1-4772-5164-5 (e)

FOREWORD

ANGLO-INDIAN CUISINE — A LEGACY OF FLAVOURS FROM THE PAST is a comprehensive and unique collection of easy-to-follow Recipes of popular and well loved Anglo-Indian dishes. The repertoire is rich and vast, ranging from the outright European Roasts, Cutlets, Croquettes, Pasties, etc, to mouth watering Curries, Side Dishes, Spicy Fries, Foogaths, Biryani and Palaus, Pickles, Chutneys etc, picking up plenty of hybrids along the way. The sumptuous Anglo-Indian dishes such as Yellow Coconut Rice and Mince Ball (Kofta) Curry / Bad word Curry, Pepper Water, Mulligatawny Soup, Grandma's Country Captain Chicken, Railway Mutton Curry, Dak Bungalow Curry, Crumbed Lamb Chops, Ding Ding, Stews, Duck Buffat, Almorth, etc, which were very popular in the olden days will take you on an exotic nostalgic journey to Culinary Paradise.

Many of the recipes in this book were given to me by my mother the late Doris White and it is from her that I developed a deep love for cooking. I have simplified the recipes so that they are easy to follow and less time consuming, besides using all common and easily available ingredients. Through trial and error I have arrived at the exact amounts of ingredients etc. to be used, besides substituting some of the ingredients to suit present day availability and health consciousness. While the basic recipe can be made use of, chicken, or vegetables can be substituted for meat and vice versa.

To get the authentic Anglo-Indian Curry taste while using the recipes in this book, use ginger and garlic paste that is ground at home in a blender using fresh root ginger and garlic. The ready made ginger and garlic paste available in stores around the world contain vinegar / acetic acid and other preservatives. These detract from the original taste of the Curry giving it a completely different flavour.

If fresh home made ginger and garlic paste is not available, then Garlic Powder can be used instead of fresh garlic. 1 teaspoon of garlic powder is equal to a whole garlic, so half a teaspoon would suffice. Ginger powder too can be substituted for fresh ginger. 1 teaspoon of dry ginger powder mixed with ¼ cup of water is equal to 2 teaspoons of fresh ginger paste, so half a teaspoon of ginger powder would be equal to 1 teaspoon of fresh ginger paste. Any good cooking oil could be used in the preparation of these dishes such as Sun flower Oil, groundnut Oil or even Olive Oil depending on one's preference.

All the Recipes in this Book are for 6 generous servings. If cooking for a smaller or larger number, the quantities should be adjusted accordingly. Likewise, the pungency of the dishes could be reduced by reducing the amount of chillie powder and other seasonings according to individual tastes.

The easy-to-follow directions make cooking these old, popular, sumptuous dishes simple, enjoyable and problem-free. I am confident that anyone who follows these recipes will turn out dishes that will truly be a gastronomic delight. **It is my hope that the recipes in this book will be a useful, if unpretentious guide to Anglo-Indian Cuisine**.

ANGLO-INDIAN CUISINE — A LEGACY OF FLAVOURS FROM THE PAST has been selected as the *'WINNER FROM INDIA'* by GOURMAND INTERNATIONAL SPAIN, *GOURMAND WORLD COOK BOOKS AWARDS 2012* under the Category: *BEST CULINARY HISTORY BOOK*

"The flavors of the past become the Culinary legacies of the future"

Bridget White

INTRODUCTION

History and Evolution of Anglo-Indian Cuisine. One of the first examples of Fusion Food in the World!!

The Word "GASTRONOMY" means "THE ART OF GOOD EATING" and this is very true of Anglo-Indian cuisine, which is an ART IN ITSELF. Anglo-Indian Cuisine is a fusion of both western and Indian Cuisine and is perhaps among the first examples of FUSION FOOD in the world.

The evolution of Anglo-Indian food makes interesting history. India was home to several European Races. Initially, the British as well as other Europeans did not relish local Indian food. Most British officers and Civil Administrators who came to India in those early years, looked upon the native cuisines of India as unhygienic and unpalatable because of the high content of spices and herbs in Indian dishes. They even hated the smell of Indian food being prepared in local kitchens. To these foreigners, whose daily diet consisted of rather bland fare, the pungent, spicy local cuisine was anathema to them.

In the early days, the British and European Memsahibs employed Indian khansamas or cooks to work for them and they taught these servants, their own cuisines rather than let them prepare Indian Fare in their homes, However, over a period of time, the cooks began adding a few local ingredients to the rather bland European food, and experimented in making puddings and sweets using local ingredients. As a result, throughout the Colonial Period many new, hybrid dishes evolved because the khansamas or cooks experimented and invented new dishes which combined some of the flavours of India with those of the West and vice versa thereby creating a new **'Anglo-Indian Cuisine'!**

During this period, Soups were seasoned with cumin and red chillies, Roasts were cooked with whole spices like cloves, pepper and cinnamon and Rissoles and Croquettes were flavored with turmeric and 'spices' Thus Curries and Sauces were invented by the Khansamas of the British to cater to their new craze for Indian 'Spice flavoured food'. Mulligatawny Soup, Meat Jalfraze (which was basically meat fried with a few spices), Tomato Ketchup etc were some of the very first innovations.

Anglo-Indian cuisine therefore evolved over many hundreds of years as a result of reinventing and reinterpreting the quintessentially western cuisine by assimilating and amalgamating ingredients and cooking techniques from all over the Indian sub-continent. Thus a completely new contemporary cuisine came into existence making it truly "Anglo" and "Indian" in nature, which was neither too bland nor too spicy, but with a distinctive flavour of its own. It became a direct reflection of the multi-cultural and hybrid heritage of the new colonial population. However, over the years, Anglo-Indian cooking became more regional oriented.

British Legacy — An Epicurean Tryst

While Anglo-Indian Cuisine could be said to be influenced by the various European invasions in India, it was the British, who actually left an indelible mark on Anglo-Indian Cuisine. Roasts, Stews, Bakes, Sandwiches and White bread are a legacy of the British, and Anglo-Indians took these to new heights, making them part of their daily cuisine. The Sunday English Breakfasts of Eggs, Bacon, Ham, Buttered Toast, Cheese, butter, Jams and the English Roast Dinners complete with steamed vegetables, Roast Potatoes, Yorkshire Pudding and gravy, English sausages, colloquially known as "bangers with mash" became part of the Anglo-Indian Culinary Repertoire.

The concept of the English High Tea in the afternoons which was a direct throw back of the Raj quickly became an Anglo-Indian custom in the early part of the century. One could conjure up images of the English and Anglo-Indian 'Memsahibs' enjoying afternoon tea laid out on tables covered with snowy white tablecloths, seated on white garden chairs on a velvet green lawn and being served tiny cucumber sandwiches, cakes, scones, butterfly cakes, and pastries by obsequious servants, and drinking tea from miniature fine Bone China teacups (all legacies of the British Raj), bringing to mind, scenes of an ordered, easy, leisurely life amid gentle Indian settings in those early times.

Scottish Influence

Just as British Cuisine was given a make over to become part of the repertoire of Anglo-Indian Cuisine with the addition of a few more ingredients to most of the dishes while still retaining the original names and the basic ingredients, many Scottish dishes too were given a slight makeover. Scottish dishes such as the Treacle Pudding, Pancakes, Scotch eggs, Short Bread, Oats Porridge, Oats and Barley and its varied uses, Beef Pepper Mince and Potatoes, (Mince and Tatties), Hotch Potch, Potato, leek and onion soup, the famous Hot toddy, Bread Pudding, Steak and Kidney pie, Cottage Pie, Washerman's Pie, Toad in the Hole, Curried sheep's head, etc are all examples of Scottish food which were given a distinctive Anglo-Indian taste. **Fish Kedgeree** was first introduced in India by the Scottish Soldiers.

The French Connection

The French left us a legacy of Baguettes, French Loaf, Croquettes, Quiches, (a variety of tarts), Crêpes, Chocolate Mousse, Éclairs, etc. Crepes became Anglo-Indian Pan Cakes and Pan Rolls with a variety of fillings such as grated coconut, minced meat and other savoury fillings. A few other French Savoury dishes that were common Anglo-Indian Fare in the olden days, are 'Coq au Vin' which locally meant 'Rooster cooked in tomatoes with a dash of Red Wine', Duck or Goose Liver Fry (Foie Gras), Crumb Fried Chicken (Poulet Goujans), etc. Besides these, the French Onion Soup, Batter fried fish, etc were other examples of French based Anglo-Indian Dishes.

Dutch Delights

The Dutch left no significant impact on Anglo-Indian Cuisine. They, however, were instrumental in introducing Baking Dough that made use of Yeast, besides, Eggs and Butter as the main ingredients along with flour. A popular item was a yeast-dough bun stuffed with curried Beef and Potatoes. Other so called Anglo-Dutch or Indo Dutch delicacies were Dutch Pancakes and 'Fricadallus' or 'Forced meat' cutlets of minced beef, chicken or fish. They also left us an enduring liking for Dutch Ball Cheese!

Portuguese Perspective

The Portuguese influence on Indian food was felt as early as 1498, when Vasco da Gama entered India. Various ingredients and condiments such as coriander, red and dried chillies, garlic, vinegar and vegetables such as potato, tomato, pumpkin, cashew nuts etc were introduced into India by the Portuguese. The Portuguese left us their famous 'Vinha De Alhos' or Vindaloo, Pickled Fish and Prawns known as Balachao, Chicken and Meat Buffards, Salted Beef Tongue, Stuffed Mackerels, Sour and Spicy Fish dishes, etc. Portuguese food makes good use of vinegar so most of these dishes have a slightly tangy taste. Sweet dishes such as Dodol, Bebinca, Kalkals, Fritters, Coconut cookies, etc are all legacies of the Portuguese.

The very popular and familiar curry dish "Vindaloo" is derived from the Portuguese word "Vinha De Alhos" i.e. from the 2 main ingredients in it, which were "Vinho", meaning wine or wine vinegar, and "Alhos", meaning garlic. It was originally a vinegar and garlic based watery stew prepared with pork or meat in Portugal. Vinegar was then substituted for wine and the dish was made more pungent with the addition of chillies and cumin. Thus was created a new "Fusion dish" which then swiftly spread and became popular throughout the country. It soon became the signature dish of the Anglo-Indian Community, and over the years it has become one of the spiciest and most popular curry dishes all over the world.

Popular Colonial Dishes

The Railway Lamb / Mutton Curry is a direct throw back to the days of the British Raj, when travelling by train was considered aristocratic. The very name 'Railway Lamb Curry conjures up scenes of leisurely travel by train in the early 1900s, of tables covered with snow white table cloths laid with gleaming china and cutlery, of turbaned waiters and bearers serving this tasty slightly tangy Curry dish with Rolls and Crusty White Bread in Railway Dining and Refreshment Rooms and in Pantry Cars on long distance trains. As its very name suggests, this very popular and tasty dish was prepared and served in Railway Refreshment Rooms and only in First Class Cabins on long distance trains, with Bread or Dinner Rolls. The curry was not too spicy keeping in mind the delicate palates of the British. It was prepared with tender pieces of lamb or mutton, potatoes and other Indian condiments along with the addition of either vinegar, tamarind juice or yogurt. The dish was left to simmer on low heat for more than an hour, so as to absorb all the flavours making it truly a dish fit for a connoisseur! It was also popular with the Anglo-Indian Railway staff, who had to be on duty for long periods at a stretch. The vinegar or Tamarind juice used in its preparation ensured that the curry would last for quite a few days and was an ideal accompaniment with rice as well.

Grandma's Country Captain Chicken was another popular dish during Colonial British times. In those days, well-fed, home grown country chickens were used in its preparation. The chickens were cooked with freshly ground ingredients over a firewood oven for hours to bring out its rich and delicious taste. This dish presumably got its name from an old Grandma who prepared this special dish for her favourite grandson, a Captain in the British Army! Another explanation is that this particular chicken dish was first prepared by a Captain on a Country Boat! Whatever the origins, it was a very popular and tasty dish that is still cooked even today in many Anglo-Indian Homes.

The Dak Bungalow Curry was a famous dish prepared by Khansamas or Cooks in Inspection or Dak Bungalows during the British Raj. It was prepared with either meat or chicken and served with rice and vegetables or bread to the British Officers when they stayed at the various Dak Bungalows, while on official trips around the country. The recipe for preparing this dish varied with each cook at the Dak Bungalows depending on the availability of ingredients in a particular place during the war. It's a well known fact that the Englishmen were quite fed up of their own bland cuisine and were always eager to sample the food cooked with Indian spices by the cooks in the various Inspection Bungalows.

The Dak Bungalow Menu in the early days usually consisted of meat or chicken (country fowls), either roasted or grilled or made into a curry, invariably served with baked potatoes, grilled tomatoes, rice kedgeree, or boiled eggs or omlettes and steamed vegetables. Since these Bungalows were situated on the main Trunk Roads with no markets or grocery shops in the vicinity, the cooks stationed at these Bungalows had to be innovative and use whatever ingredients were locally available. The Dak Bungalow recipes were therefore based more on the whims and imagination of the Cook since he had to work with primitive kitchen equipment and limited ingredients. However, as time went on, each new generation of Dak Bungalow cooks was able to obtain the recipes of the dishes by word-of-mouth from their predecessors, and being more versatile quickly picked up other cuisines as well.

Mulligatawny Soup was actually the anglicized version of the Tamil "Melligu-Thani". ("Melligu" meaning pepper and "Thani" meaning water). As the name suggests it was originally Pepper Water. However in course of time a lot of other ingredients such coconut, meat and other spices were added to give it a completely different flavour. The dish quickly became popular throughout the colonies of the Common Wealth. The Mulligatawny Soup of today bears little resemblance to the original 'MELLIGU-THANI' or our very own Anglo-Indian Pepperwater!

The Devil Curry as its name suggests, is a rich and fiery hot dish, prepared with Beef, Mutton, lamb, Chicken, Pork or Eggs and lots of chilies. In the earlier days, Wild Boar, Venison and Rabbit were also made into the Devil Curry. The Devil Curry is a modified version of the Jal Frazie that originated during the Colonial Era, where the left over Turkey and Chicken Roasts were converted into Devil Curries or Fries by giving them a makeover the next day with the addition of a few spices.

This is just a small explanation about the history of Anglo-Indian Cuisine. Thus, as a legacy of the Colonial Raj Era, we have the remnants of an Anglo-Indian, Indo-French or Indo-Portuguese cuisine. This cuisine still flourishes in parts of India and in parts of Britain, Europe, Australia and Canada where nostalgic memories of the Raj still linger on in the form of the Anglo-Indian Community. Anglo-Indian food is therefore the delicious result of the British Raj in India. Anglo-Indian Cuisine is a a gourmet's delight. It is the extremely unusual blend of tastes and the rhyming alliterative names like Pish Pash, Doldol, kalkal, Ding-Ding, Posthole, etc, that makes this cuisine so unique. The very nomenclature of the dishes is original and unique, and synonymous only to the Anglo-Indian Community which is a true reflection of both worlds.

However, due to the influences of various factors, Colonial Anglo-Indian Cuisine is slowly getting extinct. In a world fast turning into a Global Village, with many Anglo-Indians having migrated away from India and the younger generation not showing interest in our old traditional food, I felt it had therefore become imperative to preserve those very authentic tastes and flavours and record for future generations the unique heritage of the pioneers of this cuisine.

With this in mind I have brought out 5 other Cookery Books on exclusive Anglo-Indian Cuisine, with the intention of reviving and preserving for posterity, the Anglo-Indian flavours and tastes of the past, thereby preserving our Community's Culinary Heritage.

The Anglo-Indian Cookery Books published by me are listed below:

1. Anglo-Indian Delicacies
2. The Anglo-Indian Festive Hamper
3. The Anglo-Indian Snack Box
4. A Collection of Anglo-Indian Roasts, Casseroles And Bakes
5. Vegetarian Delicacies

Bridget White

CONTENTS

1. THE CURRY TRAIN
Curries, Side Dishes, Stews, Cutlets, Etc

2. Pepper Water, Soups And Mulligatawny

3. RICE DISHES — A Rendezvous' With Rice

4. Foogaths And Accompaniments

5. Anglo-Indian Pickles And Chutneys

6. SHORT CUTS AND EASIES—Some Basic Preparations

1.
THE CURRY TRAIN
CURRIES, SIDE DISHES, STEWS, CUTLETS, ETC

A. Chicken And Poultry

1. Chicken Vindaloo

Serves 6   *Preparation Time 45 minutes*

Ingredients:

1 kg chicken jointed and cut into medium pieces
3 big tomatoes pureed (optional)
2 big onions chopped
3 medium potatoes pealed and cut into quarters
3 tablespoons oil
Salt to taste
1 teaspoon powdered mustard
3 teaspoons chillie powder
2 teaspoons cumin powder
1 teaspoon pepper powder
2 teaspoons garlic paste
½ cup vinegar
½ teaspoon turmeric powder

Wash the Chicken and keep aside. Heat oil in a vessel or pressure cooker and fry the onions till golden brown. Add the garlic paste and fry well. Add the chillie powder, turmeric powder, cumin powder, mustard powder, pepper powder and a little water and fry well till the oil separates from the mixture. Add the tomato puree and salt and fry for some more time. Now add the chicken, potatoes and vinegar and mix well. Add more water depending on how much gravy is required and cook till done. (If cooking in a pressure cooker, turn off the heat after 2 or 3 whistles).

---

2. Grandma's Country Captain Chicken

Serves 6   *Preparation Time 30 minutes*

Ingredients:

1 kg chicken cut into medium size pieces
3 large onions sliced finely
2 teaspoons chillie powder
1 teaspoon turmeric powder
2 tablespoons oil
Salt to taste
2 teaspoons garlic paste
2 small sticks cinnamon
4 cloves
2 cardamoms
6 or 8 whole pepper corns
2 Dry Red Chillies broken into bits

Heat oil in a pan and fry the onions cinnamon, cloves, cardamom, red chillie and pepper corns lightly. Add the chicken, mix in the garlic paste and sauté for about 5 minutes on medium heat. Add the chillie powder, turmeric powder, and salt. Mix well and stir fry for a few minutes. Add ½ cup of water and cook till the chicken is tender and the gravy is quite thick.

Note: This recipe can be adapted to meat as well. Left over Beef or Lamb Roast can be made into a delicious County Captain Fry or a cold meat curry if desired.

3. A Simple Chicken Curry

Serves 6   Preparation Time 20 minutes

Ingredients:

1 kg chicken jointed and cut into medium size pieces
½ coconut ground to a paste or half a pack of coconut milk
A small bunch of coriander leaves washed and chopped
2 large onions chopped
½ teaspoon turmeric powder
2 or 3 teaspoons chillie powder
A few whole spices
3 teaspoons ginger garlic paste
3 tablespoons oil
Salt to taste
1 teaspoon cumin powder

Heat oil in a pan and add the onions, Fry till golden brown. Add the whole spices and ginger garlic paste and sauté for a few minutes. Now add the chicken, salt, chillie powder, turmeric powder and cumin powder and fry for some time till the oil separates from the mixture. Add the coconut and mix well. Add sufficient water and cook till the chicken is done and the gravy is thick

4. Dak Bungalow Chicken Curry

Serves 6   Preparation Time 45 minutes

Ingredients:

1 Kg chicken cut into medium size pieces
1 teaspoon spice powder or garam masala powder
3 teaspoons chopped garlic
1 teaspoon chillie powder
3 onions sliced

Salt to taste
3 green chillies
½ teaspoon turmeric powder
½ teaspoon pepper powder
2 tablespoons oil
1 tablespoon lime juice
½ cup curds / yogurt (optional)

Wash the chicken and add all the ingredients mentioned above to it and marinate for about 1 hour in a suitable pan. Place the pan on medium heat and cook closed for about 5 to 6 minutes. Lower the heat, add enough water and then simmer on low heat till the chicken is cooked and the gravy thickens.

5. Old Time Fowl Curry

Serves 6   Preparation Time 45 minutes

Ingredients:

1 medium sized fowl jointed into medium size pieces (preferably a country chicken)
2 tablespoons vinegar
3 teaspoons chopped garlic
3 onions sliced
1 tomato chopped
Salt to taste
3 tablespoons chopped coriander leaves
½ teaspoon turmeric powder
2 tablespoons chillie powder
1 tablespoon coriander powder
2 small sticks cinnamon
3 cloves
1 bayleaf
2 tablespoons oil

Marinate the chicken and with all the ingredients mentioned above for about 1 hour in a suitable pan. Place the pan on high heat and cook for about 3 or 4 minutes mixing well. Lower the heat and add 2 glasses of water. Mix well and simmer for 45 minutes till the fowl is cooked and the gravy is thick.

(If using a country fowl then cook for longer).

---

6. Rich and Spicy Chicken

Serves 6   Preparation time 45 minutes

Ingredients:

1 kg chicken cut into medium size pieces
3 onions chopped finely
2 large tomatoes chopped
2 teaspoons ginger garlic paste
1 teaspoon coriander powder
1 teaspoon poppy seeds (kus kus) optional
1 teaspoon turmeric powder
½ cup grated coconut
½ teaspoon spice powder or garam masala
Salt to taste
2 teaspoons chopped coriander leaves
2 teaspoons chopped mint leaves
3 tablespoons oil
2 teaspoons chillie powder
2 tablespoons curds

Grind the coconut, poppy seeds and half the onions to a smooth paste. Heat oil in a pan and fry the remaining onions till golden brown. Add the ground paste and fry for about 5 minutes on low heat. Add the chillie powder, ginger garlic paste, spice powder (garam masala powder), coriander powder, turmeric powder and tomatoes and keep frying till the tomatoes are reduced to pulp. Now add the chicken and curds and mix well. Add salt to taste and 2 cups of water, mint and coriander leaves and simmer till the chicken is cooked and gravy is thick. Serve hot with rice or chapattis.

---

7. Chicken Buffad (Christmas Stew)

Serves 6   *Preparation Time 45 minutes*

Ingredients:

1 kg chicken
1 large cabbage cut into 4
3 carrots cut into medium pieces
1 teaspoon turmeric powder
2 teaspoons salt
4 large onions sliced
6 green chilies slit lengthwise
1 teaspoon crushed garlic
1 teaspoon chopped ginger
½ cup vinegar
½ cup oil or ghee
1 teaspoon spice powder
2 teaspoons chillie powder
1 teaspoon pepper powder
2 Bay leaves
1 teaspoon cumin powder
2 potatoes peeled and chopped

Cut the chicken into about 8 big pieces. Wash well and add all the above ingredients to it. Mix well. Heat the oil in a large pan. Cover the bottom of the pan with the cabbage, potatoes and carrots. Add the chicken mixed with all the ingredients. Add 3 cups of water. Cover the pan and cook first on high heat then simmer on low heat for 30 minutes till the chicken pieces are well cooked and the buffad gives out a nice aroma. Serve hot.

Note: Other vegetables of your choice may used along with cabbage and carrots. This wholesome stew was a 'must have' in Anglo-Indian homes on Christmas morning in the earlier days!

8. Chicken in Thick Coconut Milk Gravy

Serves 6   Preparation Time 15 minutes

Ingredients

1 kg chicken jointed and cut into medium size pieces
A small bunch of coriander leaves washed and chopped
2 large onions chopped
2 tomatoes chopped
½ teaspoon turmeric powder
2 or 3 teaspoons chillie powder
2 cloves, 2 pieces of cinnamon, 2 cardamoms, 1 bay leaf
1 teaspoon ginger paste
1 teaspoon garlic paste
3 tablespoons oil
Salt to taste
1 teaspoon cumin powder
4 tablespoons thick Coconut milk

Heat oil in a pan and add the onions, Fry till golden brown. Add the cloves, cinnamon, cardamom, bay leaf, tomato, ginger paste and garlic paste and sauté for a few minutes. Now add the chicken, salt, chillie powder, turmeric powder and cumin powder and fry for some time till the oil separates from the mixture. Add the coconut milk and sufficient water and cook till the chicken is done and the gravy is thick

9. Chicken in Mint and Corriander Gravy

Serves 6   *Preparation time 45 minutes*

Ingredients

1 kg chicken cut into medium size pieces
3 onions chopped finely
2 large tomatoes chopped
1 teaspoon ginger paste
1 teaspoon garlic paste
1 teaspoon coriander powder
1 teaspoon turmeric powder
½ cup grated coconut
Salt to taste
2 teaspoons chopped coriander leaves
2 teaspoons chopped mint leaves
3 tablespoons oil
2 teaspoons chillie powder

Grind the coconut and half the onions to a smooth paste. Heat oil in a pan and fry the remaining onions till golden brown. Add the ground coconut and onion paste and fry for about 5 minutes on low heat. Add the chillie powder, ginger paste, garlic paste, coriander powder, turmeric powder and tomatoes and keep frying till the tomatoes are reduced to pulp. Now add the chicken and mix well. Add salt to taste and 2 cups of water, mint and coriander leaves and simmer till the chicken is cooked and gravy is thick. Serve hot with rice or chapattis.

10. Chicken in Red Wine

(A variation of Vindaloo cooked with wine instead of vinegar)

Serves 6   Preparation Time 1 hour

Ingredients

1 kg Chicken cut into medium size pieces
1 teaspoon cumin powder
3 dry red chillies broken into bits
1 teaspoon garlic and ginger paste
3 tomatoes chopped
2 onions sliced finely
1 teaspoon spice powder or garam masala powder
1 teaspoon ground pepper powder
½ teaspoon whole pepper corns
3 tablespoons oil
¾ cup red wine
Salt to taste

Heat oil in a suitable pan and add the dry red chillies, onions and pepper corns and fry till golden brown. Add the chicken and sauté for a few minutes till it changes colour. Now add all the other ingredients and stir well. Simmer on low heat till the chicken is tender and the gravy is thick. Serve with rice, chapattis or bread.

11. Chicken Stew

Serves 6   Preparation Time 1 hour

Ingredients

1 kg chicken cut into medium pieces
2 tablespoons oil
2 potatoes peeled and cut into quarters

2 carrots peeled and cut into medium size pieces
1 teaspoon pepper corns
1 tomato chopped
½ teaspoon chopped ginger
½ teaspoon chopped garlic
Salt to taste
3 green chillies slit
2 onions sliced
1 tablespoon chopped mint leaves
2 tablespoons flour

Cook the Chicken along with the potatoes, carrots, peppercorns, green chilies, tomato, ginger, garlic, mint, salt, and sufficient water till tender. Make a thin paste of the flour with about ¼ cup of water. In another pan heat the oil and fry the onions till golden brown. Add the flour paste and fry along with the onions for some time. Add the cooked chicken and potatoes and simmer for 5 minutes. Serve hot with bread or Hoppers.

12. Nana's Bobo (Fowl) Curry

Serves 6   *Preparation Time 45 minutes*

Ingredients

1 medium size chicken chopped into medium size pieces
3 onions sliced finely
2 teaspoons chopped garlic
Salt to taste
2 tablespoons chillie powder
3 tablespoons Vinegar
3 Tomatoes, chopped
2 teaspoons coriander powder
1 teaspoon cumin powder
1 teaspoon pepper powder
½ teaspoon turmeric powder
1 teaspoon chopped ginger

3 tablespoons oil
Salt to taste

Heat oil in large pan and lightly fry the chicken till brown. Remove and keep aside. In the same oil sauté the onions, chopped garlic and chopped ginger till brown. Add the chillie powder, coriander powder, cumin powder, turmeric powder, pepper powder, and tomatoes and mix well. Stir-fry for a few minutes till the tomatoes are soft. Add the chicken and vinegar and mix well. Add sufficient water and simmer on low heat till the chicken is tender and the gravy is slightly thick. Serve with Rice or Chapattis

13. Green Masala Chicken Curry

Serves 6   *Preparation time 45 minutes*

Ingredients

1 kg chicken cut into medium pieces
2-teaspoons ginger garlic paste
4 green chilies
1 cup chopped coriander leaves
1 teaspoon cumin seeds
2 cloves, 2 cardamoms, 2 pieces of cinnamon
½ teaspoon turmeric powder
Salt to taste
3-tablespoons oil
½ cup coconut paste
3 potatoes pealed washed and cut into quarters

Grind the green chilies, coriander leaves, coconut, cinnamon, cloves, cardamom and cumin seeds to a smooth paste in a blender. Heat oil in a pan and fry the onions till golden brown. Add the chicken and turmeric powder and fry for some time. Now add the ground masala and salt and mix well with the chicken. Keep frying on low heat till the oil separates from the masala. Add the potatoes and sufficient water and cook for 15 minutes of till the chicken is cooked. Serve hot.

This curry is good with ghee rice or Palau rice.

14. Colonial Pepper Chicken Fry

Serves 6   *Preparation Time 30 minutes*

Ingredients

1 kg chicken cut into medium size pieces
3 large onions sliced finely
2 teaspoons pepper powder
1 teaspoon turmeric powder
2 tablespoons oil
Salt to taste

Heat oil in a pan and fry the onions lightly. Add the chicken and mix in the pepper powder, tumeric powder and salt. Add ½ cup of water and cook on low heat till the chicken is tender and semi dry.

Note: Alternately, the chicken can be par boiled with a little water and then added to the sautéed onions and pepper.

15. Chicken Gizzards and Liver Pepper Fry

Serves 6   *Preparation Time 45 minutes*

Ingredients

½ kg chicken gizzards and liver cut into pieces
2 large onions sliced finely
2 or 3 teaspoons ground pepper
2 green chillies slit

Salt to taste
3 tablespoons oil
½ teaspoon turmeric powder

Wash the chicken gizzards and livers well. Boil them with a little water and salt till done. Heat oil in a pan and fry the onions till golden brown. Add the cooked gizzards and liver together with the slit green chillies, turmeric powder, pepper powder and salt and keep frying on low heat till dry and brown

---

16. Spicy Chicken Gizzards and Liver Fry

Serves 6   *Preparation Time 1 hour*

Ingredients

½ Kg chicken gizzards and liver cut into medium size pieces
2 teaspoons chillie powder
½ teaspoon turmeric powder
3 large onions sliced finely
½ teaspoon cumin powder
3 tablespoons oil
Salt to taste

Wash the gizzards and liver and boil them in a little water and salt till tender. Drain and keep aside, Heat oil in a pan and fry the onions till golden brown. Add the chillie powder, turmeric powder, cumin powder and the cooked gizzards and mix well. Stir fry for about 5 to 6 minutes till the gizzards are coated with the masala. Add more salt if required.

17. Crispy Fried Chicken

Serves 6   Preparation time 45 minutes

Ingredients

1 kg chicken cut into medium size pieces
2 tablespoons ginger garlic paste
2 teaspoons chillie powder
A pinch of red food coloring
Salt to taste
2 tablespoons vinegar
2 tablespoons corn flour
½ cup oil
½ teaspoon turmeric powder

Wash the chicken and marinate it with all the above ingredients (except the oil and cornflour) for 2 to 3 hours. Heat oil in a pan till smoky. Dust the chicken pieces with the corn flour and deep fry a few pieces at a time till crispy. Serve hot with onion rings and chips.

18. Dry Chicken Fry

Serves 6   Preparation Time 25 minutes

Ingredients

1 kg chicken cut into medium size pieces
2 onions sliced finely
1 teaspoon turmeric powder
2 tablespoons oil
1 teaspoon chillie powder
Salt to taste
½ teaspoon spice powder or garam masala powder

Wash the chicken and marinate it with the salt, chillie powder, turmeric powder and spice powder for about 10 minutes. Meanwhile heat oil in a pan and sauté the onions to golden brown. Toss in the marinated chicken pieces and mix well. Close the pan with a lid and cook on slow heat for about 15 minutes till the chicken is cooked. Add a teaspoon of ghee or butter and fry till all the gravy dries up and the chicken is dry. Serve with bread or pepper water and rice.

19. Green Chillie Chicken Fry

Serves 6   *Preparation Time 1 hour*

Ingredients

1 kg chicken cut into medium size pieces
1 teaspoon garlic ginger paste
1 teaspoon green chillie paste / chillie sauce
1 teaspoon Vinegar
3 tablespoons oil or butter
2 teaspoons chopped green chillies
½ teaspoon turmeric powder
1 teaspoon chopped garlic
Salt to taste

Marinate the chicken with the salt, vinegar, turmeric powder, ginger garlic paste and chillie paste / sauce and keep aside for 1 hour. Heat oil in a suitable pan and sauté the chopped garlic and green chillies for about 3 minutes. Add the marinated chicken and mix well. Stir fry for about 5 minutes till the chicken changes colour. Add a little water and simmer till the chicken is tender and the water dries up. Add one more spoon of oil or ghee and mix well. Serve with rice or bread. This can be served as a starter at parties as well.

20. Chicken Fry With Potatoes

Serves 6   *Preparation Time 45 Minutes*

Ingredients

1 chicken about 1 kg in weight cut into medium size pieces
2 potatoes boiled and cut into quarters
2 teaspoons chillie powder
1 teaspoon all spice powder or garam masala powder
2 whole red chillies
6 to 8 curry leaves
2 teaspoons chopped coriander leaves
Salt to taste
3 tablespoons oil or ghee

Wash the chicken and mix it with the chillie powder, garam masala and salt. Heat oil or ghee in a pan and add the curry leaves and red chillies. Fry for a few seconds. Add the marinated chicken and mix well. Cover and simmer on low heat till the chicken is cooked. (No water is necessary as the chicken will give out water). Keep mixing occasionally. When the chicken is tender add the boiled potatoes and mix once so that the potatoes are covered with the gravy. Garnish with chopped coriander leaves.

21. Crumbed Fried Spicy Chicken

Serves 6   *Preparation time 1 hour 20 minutes*

Ingredients

500 grams chicken cut into medium pieces with the bones
2 teaspoons chillie powder
1 teaspoon all spice powder or garam masala powder
¼ cup milk
½ cup breadcrumbs or powdered cornflakes

1 teaspoon ginger garlic paste
½ teaspoon pepper powder
Salt to taste
Oil for frying
2 eggs beaten well

Marinate the chicken with the ginger garlic paste, chillie powder, salt, milk, all spice powder / garam masala powder and pepper for 1 hour. Cook the chicken without adding water in a pan till dry. Remove from heat. Heat the oil in another suitable pan. Now dip the cooked chicken pieces in the beaten egg and coat with the breadcrumbs / crushed corn flakes. Deep fry the chicken pieces till golden brown. Serve as a snack or a side dish.

---

22. Chicken Drumsticks Fry

Serves 6   *Preparation Time 45 minutes*

Ingredients:

6 Chicken Drumsticks
3 large onions sliced finely
5 or 6 peppercorns
1 teaspoon pepper powder
1 teaspoon chillie powder
Salt to taste
1 teaspoon chopped ginger
1 teaspoon chopped garlic
2 tablespoon chopped fresh coriander
1 teaspoon chopped fresh mint
6 green chillies sliced lengthwise
3 tablespoons oil

Boil the chicken in about 1 cup of water with a little salt and the peppercorns till tender.

Heat oil in a pan and fry the onions, green chillies, ginger and garlic till golden brown. Add the boiled chicken, chillie powder and pepper powder and cook till semi dry. Stir in the chopped mint and coriander leaves and fry for a few more minutes. Serve with rice or bread.

23. Batter Fried Chicken

Serves 6   *Preparation Time 1 hour*

Ingredients

2 chickens each jointed into 4 pieces so as to get a total of 8 pieces
4 teaspoons pepper powder
Salt to taste
3 tablespoons butter
3 tablespoons oil
5 tablespoons lime juice or vinegar
3 tablespoons corn flour

Beat each chicken piece with a large knife or cleaver and then flatten with a rolling pin. Marinate the flattened chicken with the pepper powder, salt and lime juice / vinegar and keep aside for one hour.

Mix in the corn flour and one tablespoon butter. Heat a little oil in a nonstick pan and fry each chicken piece separately on medium heat till tender. When all the pieces are fried put them all back in the pan, add 2 tablespoons butter and sauté the chicken for about 5 minutes on low heat. Serve with rice or bread. (Alternately the chicken can be baked in an oven using the same recipe)

24. Chicken Cutlets

Serves 6   *Preparation Time 45 minutes*

Ingredients

300 grams chicken cut into small pieces
3 onions chopped
2 teaspoons chopped mint
1 teaspoon pepper powder
Salt to taste
2 tablespoons tomato sauce
1 teaspoon butter
1 egg beaten
3 tablespoons oil
3 tablespoons bread crumbs

Wash the chicken and cook in a little water with some salt till tender. Remove from the heat and cool. When cold, shred into very small flakes. Mix in the chopped onions, mint, pepper, salt, tomato sauce and butter. Form into oval shapes and flatten with a knife. Heat oil in a flat pan. Dip each cutlet in the beaten egg, roll in breadcrumbs then shallow fry on both sides till brown. Drain and serve with mashed potatoes and tomato ketch up.

25. Chicken Croquettes

Serves 6   *Preparation time 45 minutes*

Ingredients

3 cups boiled and shredded chicken
2 cups breadcrumbs
3 eggs beaten
3 onions chopped finely
1 tablespoon chopped mint or parsley
Salt to taste

19

1 teaspoon pepper powder
½ teaspoon spice powder (garam masala powder)
4 tablespoons oil

Heat 1tablespoon oil in a pan and sauté the onions lightly. Remove from heat then mix the chicken with the sautéed onions, breadcrumbs, mint/parsley, beaten eggs, salt, pepper and spice powder. Mix well then form into small long cigar shaped cutlets. Heat the remaining oil in a flat pan and fry the croquettes on medium heat till golden brown on both sides.

26. Whole Chicken Pot Roast

Serves 6   *Preparation Time 1 hour*

Ingredients

1 whole chicken cleaned and washed well
Salt to taste
2 teaspoons pepper powder
1 teaspoon Chillie powder
½ teaspoon turmeric powder
2 tablespoons oil or ghee

Marinate the chicken with the salt, pepper, chillie powder and turmeric powder for about half an hour. Heat oil or ghee in a thick-bottomed pan or pressure cooker and add the whole chicken. Turn the chicken from side to side and fry for about for about 5 minutes Cover the vessel with a tight lid and simmer over low heat turning the chicken occasionally till the chicken is cooked and all the water is absorbed. Continue to cook till the chicken is roasted to a lovely golden brown. Serve with roasted potatoes and boiled vegetables.

27. Pepper Chicken Roast

Serves 6   *Preparation Time 1 hour*

Ingredients

1 kg chicken jointed into fairly big pieces
2 teaspoons lime juice or vinegar
2 teaspoons chopped garlic
2 dry red chillies broken into bits
4 tablespoons Butter
Salt to taste
2 teaspoons whole pepper corns
2 onions chopped into big chunks

Heat the butter in a suitable pan and add the chicken pieces and all the other ingredients. Mix well and stir fry on high heat for a few minutes till the chicken changes colour. Add a little water and simmer on low heat till the chicken is tender and the water dries up. Keep roasting on low heat for a few more minutes till the chicken pieces are nicely browned. Serve with Mashed Potato and Bread.

28. Duck Roast

Serves 6   *Preparation Time 1 hour*

Ingredients

1 whole duck
Salt to taste
3 teaspoons pepper powder
3 tablespoons oil or ghee

Marinate the duck with the salt and pepper for about ½ an hour. Heat oil or ghee in a thick bottomed pan or pressure cooker and add the whole duck. Turn from side to side and fry for about for about 5 minutes. Add 2 cups of water. Cover the vessel with a tight lid and simmer over low heat turning the duck occasionally till it is cooked and all the water is absorbed. Continue to cook till the duck is roasted to a lovely golden brown. Serve with roasted potatoes and boiled veggies.

29. Savoury Roast Duck

Serves 6   *Preparation Time 1 hour*

Ingredients

    1 whole duck with the skin
    2 or 3 pods of garlic chopped very finely
    3 teaspoons pepper powder
    Salt to taste
    3 dried red chillies or 1 teaspoon Paprika
    2 teaspoons Tomato sauce
    2 teaspoons vinegar
    3 tablespoons oil
    3 large potatoes pealed

Rub the salt and pepper well into the duck. Heat Oil in a big Pan or Vessel and add the whole duck. Fry on high heat for about 3 minutes, turning on all sides till it changes colour. Add all the other ingredients and about 4 glasses of water and simmer till tender. Strain away any excess soup and keep aside. Add 2 tablespoons of oil or ghee and continue to simmer on low heat till the duck is nicely brown all over and the potatoes too are nicely roasted. Slice and arrange on a serving platter.

Pour the remaining soup back into the vessel and mix in 2 tablespoons of flour. Cook till the gravy thickens, stirring all the time. Spoon this gravy on top of the slices of the Duck Roast. Pour the remaining gravy on the side of the platter along with the Roast potatoes.

Alternatively the duck could be cooked in a pressure cooker till soft and then browned in a pan.

---

30. Duck Buffad

Serves 6   *Preparation Time 1 hour*

Ingredients

1 whole duck (dressed) about 1 ½ kg in weight jointed and cut into 6 or 8 big pieces
1 large cabbage cut into quarters
2 carrots cut into slices
2 potatoes peeled and cut into quarters
1 teaspoon turmeric powder
Salt to taste
4 large onions sliced
6 green chilies slit lengthwise
1 teaspoon crushed garlic
1 teaspoon chopped ginger
½ cup vinegar
3 tablespoons oil
1 teaspoon spice powder
2 teaspoons chillie powder
1 teaspoon pepper powder
2 Bay leaves
1 teaspoon cumin powder
1 teaspoon pepper corns

Take a large pan and cover the bottom with the cabbage. Add the duck and all the other ingredients. Add 4 cups of water. Cover the pan and cook first on high heat for 3 minutes, then simmer on low heat for about an hour till the duck is well cooked and it gives out a nice aroma. Serve hot with bread or Rolls.

Note: knollkol, cauliflower, carrot, radish, turnip, potato or any other vegetables could be made use of if desired.

31. Duck Vindaloo

Serves 6   *Preparation Time 45 minutes*

Ingredients

1 medium size duck jointed and cut into medium pieces
3 big tomatoes pureed
2 big onions chopped
3 medium potatoes pealed and cut into quarters
3 tablespoons oil
Salt to taste
3 teaspoons chillie powder
2 teaspoons cumin powder
1 teaspoon pepper powder
3 teaspoons garlic paste
½ cup vinegar
½ teaspoon turmeric powder

Heat oil in a vessel or pressure cooker and fry the onions till golden brown. Add the garlic paste and fry well. Add the chillie powder, turmeric powder, cumin powder, pepper powder and a little water and fry well till the oil separates from the mixture. Now add the tomato puree and salt and fry for some more time. Add the duck, potatoes and vinegar and mix well. Add more water depending on how much gravy is required and cook till done. (If cooking in a pressure cooker, turn off the heat after 8 or 9 whistles.

32. Duck Moilee

(Succulent Duck cooked with green chillies and coconut milk)

Serves 6   Preparation Time 45 minutes

Ingredients

1 tender duck jointed and cut into medium size pieces
3 big onions sliced finely
8 to 10 green chilies sliced lengthwise
2 teaspoons ginger garlic paste
1cup thick coconut milk
1 tomato chopped into 8 pieces
1 teaspoon turmeric powder
3 tablespoons oil
Salt to taste

Rub the duck all over with the turmeric powder. Heat oil in a pressure cooker or a suitable pan and lightly fry the pieces of duck. When the pieces turn light brown add all the other ingredients to it. Mix well so that all the pieces get covered. Add sufficient water and cook on medium heat till the duck is cooked and the gravy thickens. If cooking in a pressure cooker turn off the heat after 8 or 9 whistles.

33. Duck Puli Fry (Duck in Tamarind Sauce)

Serves 6   Preparation Time 1 hour

Ingredients

1 dressed duck chopped into medium size pieces (de-skin if desired)
2 big onions sliced
1 teaspoon coriander powder
4 green chillies slit lengthwise

2 teaspoons chillie powder
1teaspoon chopped ginger
1 teaspoon chopped garlic
Salt to taste
2 tablespoons oil
1 cup thick tamarind juice (add later)

Heat oil in a pressure cooker and sauté the onions lightly. Add the duck and all the other ingredients and mix well. Fry for a few minutes. Add sufficient water and pressure cook on medium heat for about 15 minutes. Open the pressure cooker and add the thick tamarind juice and mix well. Continue cooking on low heat till the gravy is thick and dark brown. Serve with Chapattis, Hoppers or Dosas

34. Christmas Turkey Roast With Stuffing

Serves 6   Preparation Time 1 hour

Ingredients

1 Whole small dressed Turkey
¼ cup vinegar
3 teaspoons pepper powder
2 cups bread crumbs
2 teaspoons dried mint powder
2 eggs beaten
1 cup of boiled peas and carrot
½ teaspoon grated lemon rind
½ cup oil
Salt to taste

Wash the turkey and rinse the insides well and keep aside. Wash the liver, heart, gizzards and other edible internal parts of the turkey well. Cook all these parts with a little water, salt and pepper powder till soft. Remove and chop into very tiny bits. This is known as the Turkey Giblets mince. Mix the cooked giblet mince with the eggs, bread crumbs, vinegar, mint powder lemon rind, salt and the boiled carrots and peas.

Now slit the turkey near the neck just above the chest and fill it well with the giblet mince mixture packing it firmly and tightly. When the turkey is stuffed well, close the opening Rub oil well all over the turkey. Place the stuffed turkey in a large vessel or pressure cooker and add sufficient water. Cook till the turkey is tender. Keep simmering till all the water dries up and the turkey turns a lovely golden brown all over. (The stuffed turkey can also be roasted in an oven if desired). Serve hot or cold with boiled vegetables and mash potatoes and Bread.

35. Left-Over Turkey Roast Devil Dry

Serves 6   *Preparation Time 1 hour*

Ingredients

Shred the left-over Turkey Roast and discard the bones
3 large onions sliced finely
2 teaspoons chillie powder
1 teaspoon turmeric powder
2 tablespoons oil
Salt to taste
1 teaspoon chopped garlic
2 sticks cinnamon
4 cloves
2 cardamoms
6 or 8 whole pepper corns
2 Dry Red Chillies broken into bits

Heat oil in a pan and fry the onions cinnamon, cloves, cardamom, chopped garlic, red chillie and pepper corns lightly. Add the shredded turkey and sauté for about 5 minutes on medium heat.

Add the chillie powder, turmeric powder, and salt. Mix well and stir fry for a few minutes. Serve with Bread or Rice.

Note; This recipe can be adapted to meat as well. Left over Chicken, Duck, Beef or Lamb Roast can be made into a delicious Devil Fry if desired.

B. Meat — Beef / Lamb / Mutton

1. Simple Beef Curry

Serves 6   *Preparation Time 1 hour*

Ingredients

1 kg tender beef cut into medium pieces
3 tablespoon's oil
2 large onions chopped finely
2 green chilies slit lengthwise
2 tablespoons ginger garlic paste
½ teaspoon turmeric powder
2 teaspoons chillie powder
2 teaspoons cumin powder
2 teaspoons coriander powder
1 teaspoon spice powder
Salt to taste
1 teaspoon chopped garlic

Boil the beef a little water, a pinch of turmeric and a little salt in a pressure cooker till tender. Heat oil in a suitable pan and sauté the onions, green chilies and the ginger garlic paste for some time. Add the chillie powder, cumin powder, coriander powder, turmeric powder, spice powder and fry for some time with a little water. Add the cooked beef along with the soup, chopped garlic and salt and simmer till the gravy is thick. Garnish with chopped coriander leaves.

2. Anglo-Indian Mince Ball Curry

(Mince Koftas in a coconut based gravy)

Serves 6   Preparation time 45 minutes

Ingredients for the Curry

3 large onions chopped
1 sprig curry leaves
3 teaspoons chillie powder
1 teaspoon coriander powder
2 teaspoons ginger garlic paste
3 big tomatoes pureed or chopped finely
½ cup ground coconut paste
1 teaspoon spice powder or garam masala
Salt to taste
3 tablespoons oil
1 teaspoon coriander leaves chopped finely for garnishing
½ teaspoon turmeric powder

Ingredients for the Mince Balls (Koftas)

½ kg minced meat either beef or mutton (fine mince)
½ teaspoon spice powder or garam masala powder
3 green chilies chopped
A small bunch of coriander leaves chopped finely
Salt to taste
½ teaspoon turmeric powder

Heat oil in a large pan and fry the onions till golden brown. Add the ginger garlic paste and the curry leaves and fry for some time. Now add the chillie powder, coriander powder, spice powder or garam masala powder, turmeric powder and coconut and fry for a few minutes till the oil separates from the mixture. Now add the tomato puree and salt and simmer for some time. Add sufficient water and bring to boil.

Meanwhile mix the spice powder, salt, chopped green chilies, turmeric powder and coriander leaves with the mince and form into small balls. When the curry is boiling, slowly drop in the mince balls carefully one by one. Simmer on slow heat for 20 minutes till the balls are cooked and the gravy is not too thick. Serve hot with Coconut Rice and Devil Chutney.

3. Anglo-Indian Meat Vindaloo

Serves 6   *Preparation Time 45 minutes*

Ingredients

½ kg beef or mutton /lamb cut into medium pieces
3 big tomatoes pureed or chopped
2 big onions chopped
3 medium potatoes pealed and cut into quarters
3 tablespoons oil
Salt to taste
1 teaspoon mustard powder
3 teaspoons chillie powder
2 teaspoons cumin powder
1 teaspoon pepper powder
3 teaspoons garlic paste
½ cup vinegar
½ teaspoon turmeric powder

Wash the meat and keep aside.

Heat oil in a vessel or pressure cooker and fry the onions till golden brown. Add the garlic paste and fry well. Add the chillie powder, turmeric powder, cumin powder, mustard powder, pepper powder and a little water and fry well till the oil separates from the mixture. Add the tomato puree and salt and fry for some more time. Now add the meat, potatoes and vinegar and mix well. Add more water depending on how much gravy is

31

required and cook till done.(If cooking in a pressure cooker, turn off the heat after 15 minutes).

4. Railway Lamb / Mutton Curry

Serves 6   Preparation Time 45 minutes

Ingredients

½ kg mutton or lamb cut into medium size pieces
6 peppercorns
2 big onions sliced
2 pieces cinnamon
2 cloves
2 cardamoms
8 to 10 curry leaves
4 red chilies broken into bits
1teaspoon chillie powder
1teaspoon ginger garlic paste
Salt to taste
2 tablespoons oil
2 tablespoons vinegar or ½ cup of tamarind juice

Wash the meat and mix it with the ginger garlic paste, salt and the chillie powder. Heat oil in a pan and fry the onions, curry leaves, red chillies and spices till golden brown. Add the meat and mix well. Fry for a few minutes. Add the vinegar / Tamarind juice and sufficient water and cook on medium heat till the meat is done. Keep frying till the gravy is thick and dark brown.

Note: Substitute beef for lamb / mutton if desired.

5. Dak Bungalow Meat Curry

Serves 6   *Preparation Time 45 minutes*

Ingredients

½ kg mutton or beef cut into medium size pieces
1 teaspoon spice powder or garam masala powder
3 teaspoons chopped garlic
1 teaspoon chillie powder
3 onions sliced
Salt to taste
3 green chillies
½ teaspoon turmeric powder
½ teaspoon pepper powder
2 tablespoons oil
1 tablespoon lime juice
½ cup curds / yogurt (optional)

Wash the meat well. Add all the ingredients mentioned above to it and marinate for about 1 hour in a suitable pan. Place the pan on medium heat and cook closed for about 5 to 6 minutes. Lower the heat, add enough water and then simmer for about 40 to 45 minutes till the meat is cooked and the gravy is thick.

6. Green Masala Meat Curry

Serves 6   *Preparation Time 1 hour*

Ingredients

½ kg beef or mutton cut into medium pieces
2 teaspoons ginger garlic paste
4 green chilies
1 cup chopped coriander leaves
1 teaspoon cumin seeds
2 cloves, 2 cardamom, 2 pieces of cinnamon

33

½ teaspoon turmeric powder
Salt to taste
3 tablespoons oil
½ cup coconut paste
3 potatoes pealed washed and cut into quarters

Grind the green chilies, coriander leaves, coconut, cinnamon, cloves, cardamom and cumin seeds to a smooth paste in a blender. Heat oil in a pressure cooker and fry the onions till golden brown. Add the meat and turmeric powder and fry for some time. Now add the ground masala and salt and mix well with the meat. Keep frying on low heat till the oil separates from the mixture. Add the potatoes and sufficient water and pressure cook for 15 minutes. Serve hot. This curry is good with ghee rice or Palau rice.

7. Tangy Meat Curry / Meat Puli Sauce

(Meat cooked with Tamarind)

Serves 6   *Preparation Time 45 minutes*

Ingredients:

½ kg mutton or beef cut into medium size pieces
2 big onions sliced
½ teaspoon coriander powder
2 teaspoons chillie powder
1teaspoon ginger garlic paste
Salt to taste
2 tablespoons oil
½ cup thick tamarind juice

Wash the meat and mix it with the ginger garlic paste, salt, coriander powder and the chillie powder. Heat oil in a pan and fry the onions till golden brown. Add the meat and mix well. Fry for a few minutes. Add sufficient water and cook on medium heat till the meat is tender. Add the thick tamarind juice and mix well. Keep frying till the gravy is thick and dark brown

---

8. Stuffed Snake Gourd Curry

Serves 6   *Preparation Time 1 hour*

Ingredients

1 kg beef or mutton mince
1 medium sized snake gourd scrape and cut into 2 inch pieces after removing the insides
3 medium sized onions chopped
3 large tomatoes pureed
½ cup coconut paste
A small bunch of coriander leaves chopped
2 teaspoons ginger garlic paste
3 teaspoons chillie powder
1 teaspoon spice powder
2 teaspoons coriander powder
½ teaspoon turmeric powder
Salt to taste
2 green chilies chopped
3 tablespoons oil

Wash the snake gourd and keep aside. Marinate the mince with a teaspoon of chillie powder, turmeric powder, a little salt and some chopped coriander leaves. In a pan heat the oil and fry the chopped onions till golden brown. Add the ginger garlic paste and sauté for some time. Add the chillie powder, coriander powder, spice powder, green chilies, coconut and salt and fry for a few minutes. Add the tomato puree and fry till the oil separates from the masala. Now add 2 cups of water and bring to boil. Meanwhile stuff the snake gourd rings with the marinated mince. Pack each ring tightly so that the mince does not fall out. Slowly drop the stuffed snake gourd pieces into the boiling curry and cook on low heat till the gravy is sufficiently thick and the mince is cooked. Garnish with chopped coriander leaves. Serve hot with coconut rice or plain rice.

---

9. Meat And Runner Beans Curry

Serves 6   *Preparation Time 1 hour*

Ingredients

½ kg meat (beef or mutton)
½ kg string beans / runner beans cut into one inch pieces
2 big onions chopped finely
3 big tomatoes pureed
2 teaspoons chillie powder
½ teaspoon turmeric powder
2 teaspoons coriander powder
2 teaspoons ginger garlic paste
½ cup coconut paste
3 tablespoons oil
Salt to taste

Heat oil in a pan or a pressure cooker and fry the onions well. Add the ginger garlic paste and sauté lightly. Add the tomato puree, turmeric powder, chillie powder and coriander powder and fry for some time. Add the meat and the beans. Mix well and continue frying for some time till the oil separates from the mixture Add salt, coconut paste and 2 cups of water. Cook till done. Serve with White Steamed Rice and a foogath.

10. Meat and Funugreek Leaves Curry

(Methi / Venthium Leaves Curry)

Serves 6   Preparation time 45 minutes

Ingredients

½ kg meat (beef or mutton)
1 cup of fenugreek / Venthium greens / Methi Greens washed well
2 big onions chopped finely
3 big tomatoes pureed
2 teaspoons chillie powder
½ teaspoon turmeric powder
2 teaspoons coriander powder
2-teaspoons ginger garlic paste
½ cup coconut paste or milk (optional)
3 tablespoons oil
Salt to taste

Heat oil in a suitable pan or pressure cooker and fry the onions well. Add the ginger garlic paste and sauté lightly. Add the tomato puree, chillie powder, turmeric powder and coriander powder and fry for some time. Add the meat and the greens and mix well. Continue frying for some time till the oil separates from the mixture and the greens shrivel up. Add salt, coconut paste and 2 cups of water and pressure cook till done.

11. Meat and Drumstick Curry

Serves 6   Preparation Time 45 minutes

Ingredients

½ kg beef or mutton / lamb cut into medium size pieces
3 or 4 tender drumsticks

2 onions chopped finely
1 teaspoon ginger and garlic paste
2 teaspoons chillie powder
1 teaspoon coriander powder
1 teaspoon cumin powder
2 medium size tomatoes chopped
2 tablespoons oil
3 tablespoons coconut paste or coconut milk
Salt to taste

Scrape the drumsticks and then cut them into 2 inch pieces. Wash and soak in a little water. Boil the meat with sufficient water and a little salt till tender. Heat oil in a pan and add the onions and fry till golden brown. Mix in the ginger garlic paste and fry for a few minutes. Add the tomatoes, chillie powder, salt, coriander powder, cumin powder and coconut paste / milk and sauté for a few minutes. Now add the drumsticks and boiled meat and mix well. Add the left over meat stock / soup or 1 cup of water and cook on low heat till the drumsticks are cooked, taking care not to overcook the drumsticks. Serve as a main curry with rice.

12. Meat And Masoor Dhal Curry

(Meat and Red lentils Curry)

Serves 6   *Preparation time 1 hour*

Ingredients:

½ kg beef or mutton cut into medium size pieces
2 medium sized onions sliced finely
½ cup Masoor dhal (Redgram dhal)
3 green chilies sliced
2 tablespoons ginger garlic paste
2 medium sized onions sliced finely
3 teaspoons chillie powder
2 teaspoons coriander powder
3 tablespoons oil

2 tablespoons ground coconut (optional)
Salt to taste
½ teaspoon turmeric powder

Heat oil in a vessel and fry the onions and green chilies for some time. Add the ginger garlic paste and fry for a few minutes. Add the meat and all the other ingredients and fry till the oil separates from the mixture. Add the coconut and dhal and mix well. Add sufficient water and cook till the meat is done. Garnish with chopped coriander leaves

13. Meat and Brinjal (Eggplant) Curry

Serves 6   *Preparation Time 1 hour*

Ingredients

½ kg meat (beef or lamb / mutton)
½ kg Brinjals / Eggplant
2 big onions chopped finely
2 big tomatoes chopped
2 teaspoons chillie powder
½ teaspoon turmeric powder
2 teaspoons coriander powder
2 teaspoons ginger garlic paste
½ cup coconut paste
3 tablespoons oil
Salt to taste

Cut the brinjals / eggplant into medium size pieces and soak in water. Heat oil in a pan or a pressure cooker and fry the onions well. Add the ginger garlic paste and sauté lightly. Add the tomatoes, chillie powder, turmeric powder and coriander powder and fry for some time. Add the meat and coconut paste. Mix well and continue frying for some time till the oil separates from the mixture Add salt and 2 or 3 cups of water and cook till the meat is tender. Add the brinjals / eggplant and mix well.

Cover and cook till the brinjals are done. Serve with White Steamed Rice and a foogath.

14. Meat And Lady's Finger / Okra Curry

Serves 6   *Preparation Time 45 minutes*

Ingredients

½ kg beef or mutton / lamb cut into medium size pieces
½ kg tender Ladyfinger / Okra
2 onions chopped finely
1 teaspoon ginger paste
1teaspoon garlic paste
2 teaspoons chillie powder
1 teaspoon coriander powder
2 medium size tomatoes chopped
2 tablespoons oil
Salt to taste

Wipe the lady's finger / okras with a dry cloth then cut them into 2 inch pieces. Discard the ends. Boil the meat with sufficient water and a little salt till tender. Heat oil in a pan and add the onions and fry till golden brown. Add the tomatoes, chillie powder, salt, coriander powder and ginger paste, garlic paste and sauté for a few minutes. Now add the lady's fingers / okra and the boiled meat and mix well. Add the left over meat stock / soup or 1 cup of water and cook on low heat till the lady's fingers / okras are just cooked, taking care not to overcook them. Serve as a main curry with rice.

15. Meat and Green Peas Curry

Serves 6　　　*Preparation Time approx 1 hour*

Ingredients

1 kg lamb /mutton or Beef cut into cubes
3 medium size potatoes, peeled and cut into quarters
1 cup green peas
1 teaspoon turmeric powder
Salt to taste
2 medium size onions finely chopped
2 tablespoons oil
1 teaspoon garlic paste
1 teaspoon ginger paste
1 teaspoon cumin powder
1 teaspoon coriander powder
½ teaspoon pepper powder
2 teaspoons chillie powder
1 tablespoon vinegar
2 Tomatoes chopped

Marinate the meat with salt and turmeric and keep aside for 10 minutes.

Heat the oil in a pan or a pressure cooker and sauté the onions for a few minutes. Add the garlic and ginger pastes and stir fry for 3 minutes. Add the marinated meat, chopped tomatoes and all the other ingredients and sauté for a few minutes. Add sufficient water, cover and simmer till the meat is tender. Then add the potatoes and peas and simmer for 5 more minutes or till the potatoes are cooked. Garnish with chopped Coriander leaves. Serve with rice.

16. Meat and Cauliflower Curry

Serves 6   Preparation Time 45 minutes

Ingredients

½ kg beef or mutton / lamb cut into medium size pieces
1 small cauliflower cut into florets
2 onions chopped finely
1 teaspoon ginger and garlic paste
2 teaspoons chillie powder
1 teaspoon coriander powder
1 teaspoon cumin powder
2 medium size tomatoes chopped
2 tablespoons oil
3 tablespoons coconut paste or coconut milk
Salt to taste
2 tablespoons chopped coriander leaves for garnishing

Soak the cauliflower florets in warm salt water for about half an hour. Heat the oil in a pan or a pressure cooker and sauté the onions for a few minutes. Add the garlic and ginger paste and stir fry for 3 minutes. Add the meat, chopped tomatoes and all the other ingredients and sauté for a few minutes. Add sufficient water and cook till the meat is tender. Then add the cauliflower florets and simmer for 5 more minutes or till tender. Garnish with chopped Coriander leaves. Serve with rice.

17. Meat and Radish Curry

Serves 6   Preparation Time 1 hour

Ingredients

½ kg meat (beef or mutton)
½ kg long white radish or the small red ones
2 big onions chopped finely

2 big tomatoes chopped finely
2 teaspoons chillie powder
½ teaspoon turmeric powder
2 teaspoons coriander powder
1 teaspoon cumin powder
2 teaspoons ginger garlic paste
½ cup coconut paste
3 tablespoons oil
Salt to taste

Scrape and cut the radish into medium size pieces. Heat oil in a pan or a pressure cooker and fry the onions well. Add the ginger garlic paste and sauté lightly. Add the tomatoes, chillie powder, turmeric powder, cumin powder and coriander powder and fry for some time. Add the meat, radish and coconut. Mix well and continue frying for some time till the oil separates from the mixture Add salt and 2 or 3 cups of water and cook till done. Serve with White Steamed Rice and a foogath.

18. Meat and Potato Korma

Serves 6   Preparation Time approx 1 hour

Ingredients

1 kg Mutton or beef cut into medium size pieces
3 medium size potatoes peeled and cut into quarters
1 cup curds / yogurt
Salt to taste
4 tablespoons chopped coriander leaves
2 tablespoons chopped mint leaves
2 teaspoons garlic paste
1 teaspoon spice powder or garam masala powder
4 green chillies
½ teaspoon turmeric powder
2 teaspoons chillie powder
2 tomatoes chopped

3 onions chopped finely
1 teaspoon cumin powder
1 teaspoon coriander powder
3 tablespoons coconut paste
3 tablespoons oil

Marinate the meat with all the above ingredients except the oil and keep aside for about one hour. Heat oil in a suitable pan and add the marinated meat. Cook on high heat for about 5 minutes mixing occasionally so that the meat does not stick to the bottom of the pan. Add 2 cups of water and the potatoes and mix well. Cover the pan and simmer on low heat till the meat is tender and the gravy is thick. Serve with Chapattis, Bread or rice.

19. Anglo-Indian Meat Pepper Fry

Serves 6   Preparation Time 45 minutes

Ingredients

½ kg Meat either Beef, Mutton or lamb
3 teaspoons fresh ground pepper
1 teaspoon chopped ginger
2 big onions sliced finely
3 tablespoons oil
3 large potatoes
Salt to taste

Wash the meat and keep aside. Wash the Potatoes, peal and cut into quarters.

Heat Oil in a pan and sauté the onions and chopped ginger for a few minutes. Add the meat, salt and pepper powder and mix well. Fry for 5 minutes on low heat turning the meat well till the pieces get firm. Add sufficient water and the potatoes and cook till done. Continue simmering on low heat till all the water is absorbed and the meat and potatoes are brown. Serve hot with bread or rice.

20. Simple Meat Fry

Serves 6   *Preparation Time approx 1 hour*

Ingredients

1 kg Beef or Mutton cut into small pieces
2 medium size onions finely chopped
2 tablespoons oil
1 teaspoon garlic paste
1 teaspoon ginger paste
1 teaspoon cumin powder
1 teaspoon coriander powder
2 teaspoons chillie powder
1 teaspoon spice powder or garam masala powder
2 Sprigs curry leaves
1 tablespoon vinegar
Salt to taste

Marinate the meat with all the above ingredients except the onions and curry leaves and keep aside for 1 hour. Heat oil in a pan and sauté the onions and curry leaves till slightly brown. Add the marinated meat and stir fry for a few minutes till the pieces become firm. Add 1 cup of water and mix well. Cover and simmer for 45 minutes or till the meat is tender and the gravy dries up. Serve as a side dish with Rice and pepper water.

21. Chillie Beef Fry

Serves 6   *Preparation time 1 hour*

Ingredients

1 kg good beef cut into medium size pieces
4 green chillies
2 capsicums / green peppers cut into strips
3 big onions sliced

1 inch piece ginger
2 pods garlic flaked
½ teaspoon pepper
2 tablespoons vinegar
Salt to taste
½ teaspoon turmeric
3 tablespoons oil

Boil the meat in a little water till tender. Keep the remaining soup aside. Grind the chillies, ginger, garlic, turmeric and pepper together and mix in the vinegar. Heat oil in a pan and fry the onions till golden brown. Add the cooked meat, ground masala and the capsicum and mix well. Add the remaining soup and cook on slow heat till the meat is brown.

---

22. Hot Beef Fry

Serves 6   Preparation Time 1 hour

Ingredients

1 kg Beef cut into cubes
3 green chillies
1 small piece cinnamon
3 onions sliced finely
1 teaspoon ginger garlic paste
1 teaspoon chillie powder
½ teaspoon turmeric powder
1 teaspoon pepper powder
2 tablespoons vinegar
Salt to taste

Boil the meat with a little salt and a pinch of turmeric in sufficient water till tender. Strain the soup and keep aside. Heat oil in a pan and sauté the onions, cinnamon and green chillies till slightly brown. Add the ginger garlic paste, chillie powder, pepper powder, turmeric powder and vinegar and fry for a few minutes. Add the meat and mix well. Add the remaining soup and keep frying till almost dry.

23. Beef Country Captain

Serves 6   Preparation Time 1 hour

Ingredients

1kg beef from the shoulder portion cut into small pieces
2 medium size onions cut finely
½ teaspoon turmeric powder
1 tablespoon garlic paste
2 teaspoons chillie powder
3 tablespoons oil
1 tablespoon butter or ghee
Salt to taste

Boil the beef in sufficient water with a little salt and a pinch of turmeric till tender. Remove from heat and cool. Mix the chillie powder, turmeric powder, salt and garlic paste with the boiled beef pieces and keep aside the soup.

Heat oil in a pan and fry the onions till golden brown. Remove from the pan and keep aside.

Now fry the marinated boiled beef in the same pan adding a tablespoon of butter or ghee and cook till the meat begins to look dry. Mix in the fried onions and simmer on low heat for 5 more minutes. Serve with rice or bread and a few steamed vegetables.

Note:*Country Captain is usually prepared with chicken. However it can be prepared with any left over cold meat as well. Hence the name Cold Meat Curry*

24. Beef and Potatoes in Tomato Gravy

Serves 6   *Preparation Time 45 minutes*

Ingredients

½ kg good beef cut into medium pieces
2 big tomatoes pureed
3 cloves, 2 pieces of cinnamon, 2 cardamoms
2 Bay leaves
1 teaspoon garlic and ginger paste
2 onions chopped
1 tablespoon chopped mint leaves
2 teaspoons chillie powder
Salt to taste
3 tablespoons oil
2 potatoes pealed and each cut into 8 pieces

Wash the meat and the potatoes. Heat oil in a pan and add the onions, cloves, cinnamon, cardamoms, bay leaves, ginger and garlic paste. Fry for a few minutes. Add the meat and the chillie powder and mix well. Keep frying on low heat for some more time. Now add the tomatoes, salt, mint leaves, potatoes, and mix well. Add sufficient water and cook till the meat is done and the gravy is thick. If cooking in a Pressure Cooker turn off the heat after 6 whistles. Serve hot with rice.

25. Shredded Beef Mash

Serves 6   *preparation Time 1 hour*

Ingredients

½ kg beef cut into medium pieces
2 large potatoes peeled and cut into quarters.
2 green chillies
1 teaspoon pepper powder

1 teaspoon cumin powder
2 tablespoons vinegar
1 teaspoon mustard powder
2 onions sliced
1 teaspoon chopped garlic
Salt to taste
2 teaspoons chopped mint

Boil the beef in sufficient water and a little salt till tender. Drain and keep the soup aside. Boil the potatoes and keep aside. Shred the meat into bits. Mix all the above ingredients together with the shredded meat and ½ cup of the left over soup. Mix in the boiled potatoes. Simmer on a low heat till the soup dries up and the mixture is semi solid. Serve with bread or Chapattis.

---

26. Lamb Hussainy Curry / Stick Curry

Serves 6   *Preparation Time 1 hour*

Ingredients

1 kg lamb or mutton cut into small cubes
1 cup curds / yogurt
1 teaspoon garlic paste
1 teaspoon turmeric powder
1 teaspoon ginger paste
2 teaspoons chillie powder
2 onions sliced
10 or 12 thick broom sticks / bamboo sticks or thin skewers 4" in length
3 tablespoons oil
Salt to taste

Marinate the meat with a little turmeric powder, salt and a little curds / yogurt for one hour.

Heat oil in a suitable vessel and sauté the onions for a few minutes. Add the ginger and garlic paste and fry for a few minutes. Add the chillie powder, turmeric powder, remaining curds and salt and stir fry for a few minutes. Add 1 cup of water and bring to boil. Meanwhile pass the broom sticks / bamboo sticks / skewers through the marinated meat. About 5 pieces should fit on each stick. Place the sticks of meat in the curry that is boiling. Close the vessel and simmer on low heat till the meat is cooked. Serve without removing the sticks. Garnish with chopped coriander leaves

27. Crumbed Lamb / Mutton Chops

Serves 6   Preparation Time 1 hour

Ingredients

1 kg lamb or mutton chops flatten them by beating
3 teaspoons pepper powder
Salt to taste
4 tablespoons bread crumbs
3 tablespoons oil
2 eggs beaten well
2 onions chopped finely
1 teaspoon chopped mint

Wash the mutton chop well and marinate them with the salt, pepper powder and mint over night or for at least 4 to 5 hours. Heat oil in a flat frying pan. Dip the chops one at a time in the beaten egg. Top with the chopped onions and cover well with bread crumbs. Shallow fry in the hot oil over slow fire. Fry each side till golden brown. Serve with wedges of lime and Tomato Sauce and Bread.

28. Pepper Lamb Spare Ribs

Serves 6   *Preparation Time approx 1 hour*

Ingredients

½ kg either lamb or Mutton Spare Ribs
1teaspoon chopped ginger
1 teaspoon chopped garlic
2 tablespoons vinegar
2 large onions sliced fine
2 or 3 green chilies sliced lengthwise
3 tablespoons oil
2 teaspoons pepper powder
Salt to taste

Wash the Spare Ribs and marinate them with the pepper powder, vinegar and salt for about 30 minutes. Heat oil in a large pan and sauté the onions and green chilies for a few minutes. Add the chopped ginger and garlic and fry for about 3 minutes. Now add the marinated spare ribs and mix well. Add sufficient water and cook till the spare ribs are tender and soft and the gravy dries up. Garnish with onion rings.

29. Green Masala Lamb / Mutton Chops

Serves 6   *Preparation Time 45 minutes*

Ingredients

½ kg lamb / mutton chops (Flatten slightly with the handle of the knife)
2 teaspoons ginger garlic paste
4 green chilies
3 tablespoons coriander leaves
1 teaspoon cumin seeds
2 cloves

2 cardamom
2 pieces of cinnamon
½ teaspoon turmeric powder
Salt to taste
3 tablespoons oil
3 potatoes pealed washed and cut into quarters
2 onions sliced finely
½ cup coconut paste

Grind the green chilies, coriander leaves, coconut, cinnamon, cloves, cardamom and cumin seeds to a smooth paste in a blender. Heat oil in a pressure cooker and fry the onions till golden brown. Add the meat, ginger garlic paste and turmeric powder and fry for some time. Now add the ground paste and salt and mix well. Keep frying on low heat till the oil separates from the mixture. Add the potatoes and sufficient water and pressure cook for 15 minutes. Serve hot. This curry is good with ghee rice or Palau rice.

30. Red Masala Lamb/Mutton Chops with Potatoes

Serves 6   *Preparation Time approx 1 hour*

Ingredients

½ kg Mutton /Lamb Chops (Flatten them)
3 or 4 potatoes, Boiled, pealed and cut in half lengthwise
4 big onions sliced
2 green chilies slit lengthwise
2 teaspoons chillie powder
2 teaspoons cumin powder
2 tablespoons vinegar
1 teaspoon garlic paste
Salt to taste
3 tablespoons oil

Marinate the chops with all the above ingredients (except the onions and potatoes) and keep aside for one hour. Heat oil in a suitable pan and sauté the onions till golden brown. Add the marinated chops and mix well. Cook the chops with sufficient water till tender letting some soup remain. Keep cooking on low heat till the soup dries up and the meat is a nice brown colour. Just before turning off the heat add the boiled potatoes and mix once so that the mixture covers the potatoes. Serve hot with bread or rice.

31. Green Chillie Lamb / Mutton Gravy Chops

Serves 6   *Preparation Time 1 hour*

Ingredients

1 Kg Mutton / Lamb Chops
2 large onions sliced finely
1 teaspoon garlic paste
2 Potatoes boiled and peeled and sliced thickly
1 teaspoon pepper powder
½ teaspoon turmeric powder
4 slit green chillies
Salt to taste
3 tablespoons oil

Wash the chops well and marinate it with the salt, pepper powder, garlic paste and turmeric powder. Cook the chops with a little water till tender. Add the onions, green chillies and oil and cook till the gravy is thick. Add the potatoes and mix lightly so that the potatoes are covered with the gravy.

32. Anglo-Indian Hot Masala Chops

Serves 6   *preparation Time 1 hour*

Ingredients

½ kg good chops either mutton, beef or veal
2 teaspoons ginger garlic paste
2 tablespoons vinegar
2 large onions sliced fine
2 or 3 green chilies sliced lengthwise
3 tablespoons oil
1 teaspoon mustard
4 cardamoms
4 cloves
2 pieces of cinnamon
1 teaspoon pepper powder
1 teaspoon chillie powder
Salt to taste
1 teaspoon cumin powder
1 teaspoon coriander powder

Roast and dry grind the mustard, cardamom, cloves and cinnamon. Wash the chops and marinate them with this ground masala powder, ginger garlic paste, pepper powder, chillie powder, vinegar, cumin powder, coriander powder and salt for about 30 minutes. Heat oil in a large pan and sauté the onions and green chilies till slightly brown. Add the marinated chops and mix well. Simmer for a few minutes. Add sufficient water and cook till the chops are done and the gravy dries up. Garnish with onion rings.

33. Boiled Lamb Chops

Serves 6   *Preparation Time 45 minutes*

Ingredients

1 kg good lamb chops with fat from the breast portion
4 onions sliced thickly
3 teaspoons pepper powder
1 tablespoon vinegar
2 tablespoons oil
Salt to taste

Marinate the chops with the pepper, vinegar, oil and salt and set aside for one hour. Place a layer of chops in a suitable non-stick pan and then arrange a layer of the thickly sliced onions on them. Arrange as many layers of the chops and onions in this way. Pour the remaining marinade over the chops. Close the pan with a tight fitting lid. Simmer on low heat for about 2 hours (shaking the pan gently occasionally) till the chops are tender. No water is required to be added as the meat will cook in its own juice. Since the gravy will be purely of the meat it will taste delicious.

The same recipe could be used for beef and veal chops as well

34. Dry Pepper Beef Chops

Serves 6   *Preparation time 1 hour*

Ingredients

½ kg good beef chops
2 large onions sliced
2 or 3 green chilies sliced lengthwise
3 tablespoons oil
2 teaspoons pepper powder
3 potatoes peeled and halved

Wash the chops and marinate them with the pepper powder, and salt for about 30 minutes. Heat oil in a large pan and sauté the onions and green chilies for a few minutes. Add the marinated chops and mix well. Simmer for a few minutes till the chops get firm. Add sufficient water and the potatoes and cook till the chops are done and the gravy dries up. Garnish with onion rings.

35. Beef Ding-Ding (Savoury Sun Dried Meat Crispies)

Serves 6   Preparation Time 45 minutes

Ingredients

1 kg beef from the shank end of the leg (cut into very thin slices)
3 or 4 teaspoons pepper powder
2 teaspoons chillie powder
3 teaspoons salt
1 teaspoon turmeric powder
½ cup vinegar

Wash the meat and marinate with the pepper powder, salt, chillie powder, vinegar and turmeric powder for 2 or 3 hours. String the pieces of meat on a string and hang to dry. (Alternately the marinated meat could be placed on a flat plate and kept in the sunlight to dry). The pieces should be dried thoroughly. Store in an airtight container and use whenever required at a later date.

To use at a later date, soak the dried meat pieces in cold water for a couple of hours. Beat each piece with a rolling pin and then shallow fry with a little oil. This goes well with rice and pepper water.

36. Jerky Beef (Another Version of Ding Ding)

Serves 6   *Preparation Time 1 hour*

Ingredients

1 kg tender Beef sliced thinly into 2" strips
3 teaspoons chillie powder
1 teaspoon turmeric powder
2 tablespoons vinegar
3 teaspoons salt
4 tablespoons oil

Wash the meat and dry well. Jerk or pull the pieces so that they stretch. Marinate these meat strips with the chillie powder, turmeric powder, vinegar and salt for about 3 hours. Heat oil in a frying pan and shallow fry the marinated meat pieces on medium heat till brown and crispy.

37. Green Masala Veal Curry

Serves 6   *Preparation time 45 minutes*

Ingredients

½ kg veal cut into medium size pieces
2 teaspoons ginger garlic paste
4 green chilies
1 cup chopped coriander leaves
1 teaspoon cumin seeds
2 cloves, 2 cardamom, 2 pieces of cinnamon
½ teaspoon turmeric powder
Salt to taste
3 tablespoons oil
½ cup coconut paste
3 potatoes pealed washed and cut into quarters

Grind the green chilies, coriander leaves, coconut, cinnamon, cloves, cardamom and cumin seeds to a smooth paste in a blender. Heat oil in a pressure cooker and fry the onions till golden brown. Add the Veal and turmeric powder and fry for some time. Now add the ground masala and salt and mix well. Keep frying on low heat till the oil separates from the masala. Add the potatoes and sufficient water and pressure cook for 15 minutes. Serve hot. This curry is good with ghee rice or Palau rice.

38. Spicy Veal Curry

Serves 6   Preparation Time 40 minutes

Ingredients:

1 kg very tender veal cut into medium pieces
2 large onions chopped
1teaspoon chillie powder
½ teaspoon pepper powder
½ teaspoon turmeric powder
2 tablespoons oil
1 teaspoon finely chopped ginger
2 teaspoons finely chopped garlic
Salt to taste
2 green chillies slit lengthwise
1 teaspoon cumin powder
½ teaspoon coriander powder
1 teaspoon spice powder

Wash the veal well. Cook it in sufficient water with a little salt in a suitable pan or pressure cooker till soft. Drain and keep the soup aside. Heat the oil in a pan and sauté the onions lightly. Add the veal, ginger, garlic, salt, turmeric powder, chillie powder, cumin powder, coriander powder, spice powder and pepper powder and mix well. Add the soup. Cover and simmer on low heat till the gravy thickens. Serve hot with rice or bread.

(This recipe can be used while cooking Kutty Pie as well)

---

39. Veal And Potato Korma

Serves 6   Preparation Time 45 minutes

Ingredients

½ kg good veal cut into medium pieces
2 big tomatoes pureed
1 cup curds (yogurt)
1 teaspoon spice powder (garam masala)
½ cup coconut paste
2 tablespoons ginger garlic paste
1 tablespoon chopped mint leaves
2 teaspoons chillie powder
Salt to taste
3 tablespoons oil
2 potatoes pealed and each cut into 8 pieces

Wash the meat and the potatoes. Heat oil in a pan and add the ginger garlic paste. Fry for some time. Add the meat and the chillie powder and mix well. Keep frying on low heat for some more time. Now add the tomatoes, curds, salt, mint leaves, potatoes, spice powder and the coconut and mix well. Add sufficient water and cook till the meat is done and the gravy is thick. Serve hot with rice.

---

40. Veal Vindaloo

Serves 6   Preparation time 1 hour

Ingredients

1 kg Veal cut into medium pieces
3 big tomatoes pureed

2 big onions chopped
3 medium potatoes pealed and cut into quarters
3 tablespoons oil
Salt to taste
1 teaspoon mustard powder
3 teaspoons chillie powder
2 teaspoons cumin powder
1 teaspoon pepper powder
3 teaspoons garlic paste
½ cup vinegar
½ teaspoon turmeric powder

Heat oil in a pan or pressure cooker and fry the onions till golden brown. Add the garlic paste and fry well. Add the chillie powder, turmeric powder, cumin powder, mustard powder, pepper powder and a little water and fry well till the oil separates from the mixture. Now add the tomato puree and salt and fry for some more time. Add the veal, potatoes and vinegar and mix well. Add more water depending on how much gravy is required and cook till done. (If cooking in a pressure cooker, turn off the heat after 4 or 5 whistles).

41. Savory Veal Fry

Serves 6   *Preparation Time 45 minutes*

Ingredients

½ kg tender Veal cut into medium pieces
1 big tomato chopped
2 large onions sliced finely
2 green chilies sliced lengthwise
2 teaspoons ginger garlic paste
2 tablespoons oil
1 teaspoon chillie powder
½ teaspoon turmeric powder
Salt to taste

Wash the meat and cook it together with the tomato, turmeric and salt. Let a little soup remain. Add the chillie powder, green chilies, sliced onions and ginger garlic paste and cook on low heat till the soup dries up. Add the oil and keep on frying on low heat till the meat turns brown.

42. Veal Pepper Chops

Serves 6   *Preparation Time 45 minutes*

Ingredients

½ kg good veal chops (Flatten them)
3 or 4 potatoes (Boil peal and cut each in half lengthwise)
4 big onions sliced
2 green chilies slit lengthwise
2 teaspoons pepper powder
Salt to taste
3 tablespoons oil

Cook the veal chops with a little water in a suitable pan or pressure cooker till tender letting some soup remain. Add the onions, green chilies, salt, pepper powder and oil and mix well. Keep cooking on low heat till the soup dries up and the onions and meat are a nice brown. Just before turning off the heat add the boiled potatoes and mix once so that the gravy covers the potatoes. Serve hot with bread or rice as a side dish.

43. Brown Stew (Meat And Vegetable Stew)

Serves 6   *Preparation Time 1 hour*

Ingredients

½ kg beef or mutton cut into medium pieces
3 carrots, 4 French beans, ½ cauliflower, 2 potatoes,

61

½ cabbage, washed and cut into medium pieces
4 green chilies slit lengthwise
2 medium size tomatoes chopped
1 big onion sliced
2 teaspoons ginger garlic paste
2 cloves, 2 pieces of cinnamon
6 or 7 pepper corns
A few mint leaves
Salt to taste
2 tablespoons oil
2 tablespoons coconut paste (optional)
2 tablespoons flour

Cook the vegetables and meat together with the pepper corns, green chilies, tomatoes ginger garlic paste, salt, cinnamon, cloves, mint and coconut in sufficient water till the meat is cooked. Make a thin paste of the flour and about ¼ cup of water. In another pan heat the oil and fry the onions till golden brown. Add the flour paste and fry along with the onions for some time. Now add the cooked meat and vegetables and simmer for 5 minutes. Serve hot with bread or hoppers.

Note: For Dumpling Stew, make dumplings as follows and add along with the meat and vegetables while cooking.

To make the dumplings, you will need 1 cup of flour, 1 teaspoon butter and a pinch of salt. Mix all together with a little water to form soft dough. Form into small balls and flatten slightly. Add to the stew while cooking.

---

44. Almorth (Mixed Meat And Vegetable Stew)

This dish is a kind of stew made with a combination of meat, chicken, pork and vegetables. It's a very old Anglo-Indian recipe. However, any combination of meat could be used as per personal preference. The same recipe could be used with chicken only. This Stew was a must have for Christmas Breakfast in

almost all Anglo-Indian Homes in the olden days and was eaten with bread or rolls.

Serves 6   *Preparation Time 1 hour*

Ingredients

¼ kg Beef
¼ kg mutton / lamb
½ kg chicken
¼ kg pork
A few carrots and beans chopped into medium size pieces
(or any other English vegetables)
3 potatoes peeled and cut into quarters
2 teaspoons chillie powder
½ teaspoon turmeric powder
2 teaspoons pepper powder
1 teaspoon coriander powder
4 dry red chillies broken into pieces
2 teaspoons chopped garlic
2 pieces cinnamon
5 cloves
3 onions sliced
2 tomatoes chopped
2 tablespoons chopped mint
3 tablespoons oil
Salt to taste
2 tablespoons coconut paste
2 tablespoons vinegar

Cut the meat, chicken and pork into small pieces. Heat oil in a pressure cooker or a suitable vessel and add the onions, cinnamon, cloves and chopped garlic. Fry till the onions turn golden brown. Add the mutton, beef, chicken and pork together with the chillie powder, turmeric powder, pepper powder, salt coriander powder and tomatoes and mix well. Fry till the tomatoes turn to pulp. Add the broken dry red chillies, mint and the coconut paste and mix well. Add sufficient water and cook till the meat is soft. If cooking in a pressure cooker, cook for 10 minutes (6 to 8 whistles). Now add the chopped vegetables and vinegar and simmer on low heat till the vegetables are cooked and the gravy is thick. Serve with rice, chapattis or bread.

---

45. Meat Coconut Stew

Serves 6   *Preparation Time approx 1 hour*

Ingredients

1 kg Beef or Mutton / Lamb cut into cubes
2 tablespoons oil
2 onions sliced finely
1 Bay leaf
4 or 5 cloves
6 or 8 peppercorns
3 cardamoms
2 pieces cinnamon
1 teaspoon garlic paste
1 teaspoon ginger paste
2 teaspoons flour
2 tomatoes chopped or pureed
2 carrots peeled and cut into pieces
2 potatoes peeled and cut into cubes
1 cup cauliflower florets
½ cup beans cut into 1 inch pieces
3 green chillies slit
2 tablespoons coconut paste (optional)
Salt to taste

Heat the oil in a pressure cooker or suitable pan. Add all the whole spices and fry lightly. Add the onions and fry till golden brown. Add the ginger paste, garlic paste and green chillies and fry for a few minutes. Add the tomato and fry till the oil separates. Now add the meat and stir fry for 5 more minutes. Next add the cut vegetables, coconut paste, salt and sufficient water and cook on high heat for 10 minutes. Release the steam and open the pressure cooker. Now add the flour mixed with a little water and mix well. Simmer for a few more minutes. Serve hot with Rice or bread.

---

46. Stewed Kidneys

Serves 6   *Preparation Time 45 minutes*

Ingredients:

10 lamb kidneys or 1 calf kidney
4 small onions sliced finely
2 teaspoons pepper powder
Salt to taste
2 tablespoons oil

Wash and clean the kidneys and cut into small slices.

Heat the oil in a pan and sauté the onions lightly. Add the kidney pieces, salt and pepper and mix well. Add 1 cup of water and cook on low heat till the kidneys are cooked. Thicken the gravy with a tablespoon of flour mixed with a little water. This dish goes well with toast and baked beans.

---

47. Lamb Kidneys and Potato Stew

Serves 6   *Preparation Time 30 minutes*

Ingredients

6 or 8 sheep kidneys cut into halves or 1 Beef kidney cut into bits
2 medium onions chopped
2 green chillies slit lengthwise
1 teaspoon chopped garlic

1 teaspoon peppercorns
2 potatoes peeled and cut into thin strips
Salt to taste
2 tablespoons oil

Wash the kidneys and remove the white skin. Heat oil in a pan and add the kidneys along with all the other ingredients in the raw state. Mix well and stir fry for a few minutes. Add 1 cup of water and simmer till the kidneys and potatoes are cooked. Add a tablespoon of flour and thicken the stew. Serve hot with Bread.

48. Beef Posthole Mince

Serves 6   *Preparation Time 45 minutes*

Ingredients

½ kg beef mince
2 big onions chopped
½ teaspoon turmeric powder
1 teaspoon chopped garlic
1teaspoon chopped ginger
3 green chilies chopped finely
1 small bunch coriander leaves
2 tablespoons oil
Salt to taste
½ teaspoon chillie powder

Heat oil in a pan and fry the onions till golden brown. Add the chopped ginger, garlic, green chilies, turmeric powder, chillie powder and sauté for 3 minutes. Add the mince and salt and mix well. Add the chopped coriander leaves and cook on low heat for about ½ an hour till the mince is cooked and all the water evaporates. Simmer on low heat till the mince gives out a nice aroma. Serve hot with bread or chapattis.

49. Pepper Mince Fry

Serves 6   *Preparation Time 45 minutes*

Ingredients

½ kg Mince (Beef or Mutton)
2 big Onions chopped
½ teaspoon turmeric powder
1 teaspoon chopped garlic
2 green chilies chopped finely
2 tablespoons oil
Salt to taste
2 teaspoons pepper powder
2 Potatoes boiled and chopped into small pieces

Heat oil in a pan and fry the chopped garlic and onions till golden brown. Add the green chilies, turmeric powder, pepper powder and sauté for 3 minutes. Add the mince and salt and mix well. Cook on low heat for about ½ an hour till the mince is cooked and all the water evaporates. Add the Potatoes and mix well. Simmer on low heat for 3 more minutes. Serve hot with bread or chapattis.

50. Mince and Green Peas

Serves 6   *Preparation time 30 minutes*

Ingredients:

½ kg mince (beef, mutton, pork or lamb)
2 onions chopped
1 large tomato chopped
2 green chilies chopped
2 teaspoons chopped garlic
1 teaspoon cumin powder
½ teaspoon turmeric powder

Salt to taste
2 teaspoons chillie powder
2 tablespoons chopped coriander leaves
2 tablespoons oil
½ cup green peas

Heat oil in a pan and sauté the onions, chopped garlic and green chilies. Add the mince and fry for some time. Now add the chillie powder, cumin powder, chopped tomato, turmeric powder and salt and keep on frying till the mince is firm. Add the green peas and sufficient water for gravy and cook on low heat till the gravy is thick and mince is cooked. Garnish with chopped coriander leaves. (A little ground coconut can be added if thick gravy is required).

Note. Chopped cabbage, chopped carrot, cauliflower, fenugreek / methi / venthium greens etc can be substituted for the green peas.

51. Stewed Meat Balls

Serves 6   Preparation Time approx 1 hour

Ingredients

1 kg Beef or Mutton Mince
3 onions chopped finely
3 tablespoons chopped coriander leaves or chopped parsley
2 teaspoons chillie powder
1 teaspoon pepper powder
4 tablespoons breadcrumbs
2 tablespoons tomato sauce
2 tablespoons flour
Salt to taste
4 tablespoons oil

Mix the mince with the chopped onions, coriander leaves / parsley, chillie powder, pepper powder, salt and bread crumbs and set aside for one hour. Squeeze out all the water. Divide into equal size portions then roll into balls. Heat oil in a nonstick pan and fry the meat balls gently till they are brown. Remove and keep aside.

In the same oil add 2 tablespoons of flour, 1 teaspoon pepper powder, a pinch of salt and 2 tablespoons tomato sauce and mix well. Add 1 cup of water and bring to boil.

Add the fried meat balls and shake the pan gently so that the gravy covers all of them. Simmer on low heat for about 20 minutes till the meat balls are firm. The gravy will be quite thick. Serve with bread or Pilaf rice.

52. Anglo-Indian Savoury Mince Cutlets

Serves 6 *Preparation Time 1 hour*

Ingredients

½ kg fine beef or lamb mince
1 teaspoon chopped ginger and garlic
1 medium sized onion chopped finely
2 green chilies chopped finely
1 teaspoon pepper powder
Salt to taste
A few mint leaves chopped or ½ teaspoon mint powder
3 tablespoons oil
1 egg beaten
2 tablespoons breadcrumbs
3 large potatoes

Boil the potatoes, remove the skin and mash well. Keep aside. In a pan add the mince, ginger, garlic, onions, mint, green chilies, pepper powder and salt with a little oil and cook till the mince is dry. Remove from heat and cool for some time. Mix it well with the potatoes. Form into oval or round shaped cutlets, flatten and dip in the beaten egg then roll in the breadcrumbs. Heat the oil in a flat pan and shallow fry the cutlets on low heat till golden brown on both sides.

53. Mince Potato Chops (Pepper Mince and Potato Cutlets)

Serves 6   *Preparation Time 1 hour*

Ingredients

½ kg finely minced meat
1 medium sized onion chopped finely
2 teaspoons pepper powder
Salt to taste
3 tablespoons oil
1 egg beaten
2 tablespoons breadcrumbs
3 large potatoes

Boil the potatoes, remove the skin and mash well. Keep aside. In a pan add the mince, onions, pepper powder and salt with a little oil and cook till the mince is dry. Remove from heat and cool for some time. Form the mashed potatoes into even sized balls. Make a depression in the center and fill with the pepper mince. Flatten each ball to form a round cutlet. Dip in the beaten egg then roll in the breadcrumbs. Heat oil in a flat pan and shallow fry the cutlets on low heat till golden brown on both sides.

54. Meat Croquettes

Serves 6   *Preparation Time 45 minutes*

Ingredients

300 grams meat either beef or mutton cut into small pieces
3 onions chopped
2 teaspoons chopped mint
1 teaspoon pepper powder
Salt to taste
2 tablespoons tomato sauce
1 teaspoon butter
1 egg beaten
Yolk of one egg
3 tablespoons oil
3 tablespoons bread crumbs

Wash the meat and cook in a little water with some salt till soft. Remove from the heat and cool. When the meat is cold, shred into very small flakes. Mix in the chopped onions, mint, pepper, salt, sauce, butter and the egg yolk. Form into oval shapes and flatten with a knife. Heat the oil in a flat pan. Dip each croquette in the beaten egg, roll in bread crumbs then shallow fry on both sides till brown.

Drain and serve with mashed potatoes.

Note: Left over Roast meat can also be made into delicious Croquettes

55. Beef Mince Croquettes

Serves 6   *Preparation Time 1 hour*

Ingredients

½ kg Beef mince
I onion chopped finely
6 cloves garlic chopped
3 green chilies chopped finely
2 slices bread soaked in water and squeezed dry
3 tablespoons bread crumbs
2 eggs beaten separately
Salt to taste
3 tablespoons oil or ghee
½ teaspoon pepper powder
1 teaspoon chopped coriander and mint leaves

Wash the mince well and then cook it along with the chopped onion, green chilies, garlic, salt and a little water till nice and dry. Mix in the soaked bread slices, pepper, coriander leaves, 2 teaspoons breadcrumbs and 1 beaten egg and mix well. Form into long cigar shaped cutlets. Dip each Croquette in the remaining beaten egg and roll in breadcrumbs. Heat oil in a flat pan and shallow fry about 6 Croquettes at a time, till nicely browned all over. Serve hot with wedges of lemon and onion rings. This is a very nice accompaniment with pepper water and white rice.

56. Lamb /Mutton Mince Cutlets

Serves 6   *Preparation Time 1 hour*

Ingredients

1 kg Beef or Mutton Mince
2 large onions sliced finely
2 green chillies chopped finely

3 tablespoons oil
1 teaspoon garlic paste
1 teaspoon ginger paste
1 teaspoon cumin powder
1 teaspoon coriander powder
1 teaspoon chillie powder
1 teaspoon spice powder or garam masala
½ teaspoon nutmeg powder (Optional)
1 teaspoon finely chopped coriander leaves
3 tablespoons breadcrumbs or Semolina
1 egg beaten
Salt to taste

Cook the mince with the onions, a little salt, ginger and garlic paste and a little water till tender and dry. Remove from heat then mix in all the above ingredients except the oil and Egg. Form into cutlets. Dip each cutlet in the beaten egg covering it all over. Roll in the breadcrumbs / semolina. Heat the oil in a flat pan and shallow fry the cutlets till brown on both sides. Serve with Bread or as a snack with chips and salad.

57. Fricadels (Dutch Forced Meat Cutlets)

Serves 6   *Preparation Time 45 minutes*

Ingredients

½ kg Minced beef
3 large potatoes boiled and peeled and mashed
½ teaspoon ground cinnamon
1 teaspoon garlic paste
2 onions chopped finely
1 teaspoon black ground pepper powder
1 tablespoon vinegar
1 tablespoon chopped fresh mint leaves (or dry mint)
2 green chillies finely chopped
2 tablespoons flour

2 eggs beaten
4 tablespoons breadcrumbs
Oil for deep frying
Salt to taste

Heat 2 tablespoons oil in a suitable pan and sauté the onions for about 2 minutes. Add the mince, salt, pepper, cinnamon, garlic paste, mint, green chillies and vinegar and cook on medium heat till the mince is cooked and dry. Remove the pan from the heat, and allow the cooked mince to cool. When cold, mix the cooked mince with the mashed potato.

Heat sufficient oil in frying pan for deep frying. Using floured hands, make small lemon sized balls with the mince and potato mixture. Dip each meat ball in the beaten eggs, then roll in breadcrumbs and deep fry the mince balls till golden brown. Serve as a side dish or as a snack with tomato ketchup or mint chutney.

58. Spicy Meat Patties

Serves 6   *Preparation Time 45 minutes*

Ingredients

½ kg beef or mutton cut into small pieces.
2 tablespoons Bengal gram or channa dhal
A few mint leaves or ½ teaspoon mint powder
3 tablespoons oil
3 green chilies
1 teaspoon pepper powder
1 tablespoon chopped coriander leaves
Salt to taste

Cook the mince with all the above ingredients and a little water till the meat is tender and the water dries up completely. Keep aside to cool for some time. Grind roughly in a blender. Form into small round cutlets. Heat oil in a flat pan and shallow fry the cutlets till brown on both sides. Serve with bread or rice and pepper water

---

59. Brinjal Bake / Stuffed Brinjals

(Stuffed Eggplant / Aubergine Bake)

Serves 6   *Preparation Time 1 hour*

Ingredients

½ kg beef or mutton mince
6 big seedless Brinjals / Eggplants
4 Tablespoons oil
1 big onion sliced finely
1 tomato chopped finely
1 tablespoon flour
1 teaspoon salt
1 teaspoon pepper powder
4 green chilies chopped finely
2 tablespoons garlic chopped finely
2 eggs beaten well
4 tablespoons breadcrumbs or semolina

Wash the brinjals / eggplants and put them whole into boiling water with ½ teaspoon salt and cook for about 5 minutes till they are half cooked. Cut the brinjals into halves lengthwise dividing even the stalks. Scoop out the insides and keep aside.

Heat 2 tablespoons oil in a pan and add the onions, mince, tomato, salt, pepper, green chilies, garlic and cook on low heat till the mince is cooked and all the water is absorbed. Add the cooked insides of the brinjals and mix well. Keep aside to cool for some time. When slightly cold, fill this cooked mince in the scooped out brinjal halves and press well. Coat with the beaten egg and sprinkle the breadcrumbs or semolina on the top. Brush the sides with oil and place in a baking tray. Drizzle the remaining oil all over the stuffed brinjals and bake in a hot oven for about 15 minutes. Serve hot with bread and chips. The stuffed bringals could also be shallow fried like cutlets instead of baking

---

60. Pasties (Cornish Pasties)

Serves 6   *Preparation time 2 hours (including baking)*

Ingredients

For the Filling:
4 medium size potatoes
2 onions chopped
½ kg beef from the round portion (or mutton) cut into small bits
2 teaspoons pepper
Salt to taste
1 teaspoon chopped mint
For the Pie Crust Dough
3 cups flour
3 tablespoons oil
2 teaspoons butter
½ cup water or just enough to make a soft dough

Pre heat oven to 350°. Wash and peel the potatoes and cut into small cubes. Wash the meat well. Mix the potatoes, chopped onions, mint, meat, salt and pepper together and fry lightly with a little oil on low heat for about 5 to 6 minutes. Keep aside. This is the filling for the Pasties.

Mix flour and the oil and just enough water to make a soft pie crust dough. Roll out dough into 6 equal circles using a saucer to cut them. In the center of each circle spoon in the filling utilizing all the filling for the 6 Pasties. Put a tablespoon of butter over each mound of filling. Fold the circle over and crimp the edges.

Place pasties on a greased baking tray and make a slit in the top of each. Bake for about one hour till done.

---

61. Spicy Liver and Onion Fry

Serves 6   *Preparation Time 40 minutes*

Ingredients

½ kg beef or lamb liver sliced thinly
4 large onions sliced
1 teaspoon chillie powder
1 teaspoon pepper powder
½ teaspoon turmeric powder
2 tablespoons oil
1 teaspoon ginger garlic paste
Salt to taste
1 teaspoon cumin powder
½ teaspoon coriander powder

Wash the liver well. Heat the oil in a pan and sauté the onions lightly. Add the sliced liver, ginger garlic paste, salt turmeric powder, chillie powder, cumin powder, coriander powder and pepper powder and mix well. Cover and simmer on low heat till the liver is cooked. Add a little water while cooking if gravy is required. Serve hot with rice or bread.

---

62. Tripe — Hot and Spicy

Tripe or Boty Curry was a very popular Anglo-Indian dish. In the olden days it was prepared with freshly roasted and pounded ingredients. The Boty or the Tripe was washed well and cut into long thin strips then cooked in sufficient water for hours till tender over a firewood oven. Some people added Bengal Gram Dhal to it to make the curry thicker. Now with a pressure cooker the same dish can be prepared in

77

just 45 minutes. It is served with bread or rice and sometimes as an accompaniment with drinks. Tripe tastes delicious with Coconut Rice.

Serves 6   Preparation Time 40 minutes

Ingredients

1 kg Tripe either beef or mutton sliced thinly
2 large onions chopped
2 teaspoons chillie powder
½ teaspoon turmeric powder
2 tablespoons oil
1 teaspoon finely chopped ginger
2 teaspoons finely chopped garlic
Salt to taste
2 green chillies slit lengthwise
1 teaspoon cumin powder
½ teaspoon coriander powder

Wash the tripe well. Cook it in sufficient water and a little salt in a suitable pan or a pressure cooker till soft. Drain and keep the soup aside. Heat the oil in a pan and sauté the onions, chopped ginger and garlic lightly. Add the cooked tripe, salt, turmeric powder, chillie powder, cumin powder, coriander powder and mix well. Add the soup. Cover and simmer on low heat till the gravy thickens. Serve hot with rice or bread.

NOTE: The same recipe could be followed while preparing KUTTY PI

63. Ox Tongue Vinaloo

Serves 6   *Preparation time 45 minutes*

Ingredients

1 whole Ox tongue
3 onions chopped
2 teaspoons cumin powder
1 teaspoon turmeric powder
3 teaspoon chillie powder
1 teaspoon pepper powder
2 teaspoons garlic paste
1 cup vinegar
3 tablespoons oil
Salt to taste

Cook the tongue till soft with sufficient water. Cool and remove the white skin. Cut into slices. Heat oil and fry the onions till golden brown. Add the garlic paste and sauté for some time. Add the chillie powder, cumin powder, turmeric powder, pepper powder and fry well with a little vinegar. Continue frying till the oil separates from the masala. Add the remaining vinegar and the cooked Oxtail together with the remaining soup and cook till the gravy is thick. Serve hot with rice or bread or even hoppers.

64. Braised Ox Tongue / Ox Tongue Glaze

Serves 6   *Preparation Time approx 1 hour*

Ingredients

1 Ox Tongue
2 onions sliced
2 Carrots peeled and diced
1 teaspoon coriander powder
1 teaspoon chillie powder

½ teaspoon nutmeg powder (optional)
3 tablespoons Oil
Salt to taste

Wash the Ox Tongue and boil it in salted water till tender. Cool then slice it.

Heat oil in a pan and sauté the onions till slightly brown. Add the carrots, chillie powder, coriander powder, nutmeg powder, a little salt and about 4 tablespoons of the tongue stock and cook till the carrots are soft. Mash the carrots well. Now add the cooked slices of Ox Tongue and the remaining stock. Mix well and simmer on low heat for about 10 minutes. Serve with Bread or with rice.

65. Trotters in Gravy

Serves 6   *Preparation Time 1 hour*

Ingredients

8 Trotters either lamb or goat preferably the front ones
2 large tomatoes pureed
3 teaspoons chillie powder
2 large onions chopped
1 teaspoon ginger garlic paste
1 teaspoon coriander powder
3 tablespoons oil
Salt to taste
A small bunch of coriander leaves chopped.

Wash the trotters well and cook with sufficient water and a little salt in a pressure cooker till soft.

Heat the oil in a pan and lightly sauté the onions. Add the cooked trotters, ginger garlic paste, chillie powder, coriander powder, tomato puree and mix well. Cook first on high heat then on low heat for half an hour till the trotters are well cooked. Garnish with chopped coriander leaves. Serve hot with rice or bread or even dosas or hoppers.

---

66. Trotters in a Tangy Gravy (Trotters Puli Fry)

Serves 6   Preparation time 45 minutes

Ingredients

8 Trotters
2 big onions sliced
1 teaspoon coriander powder
4 green chillies slit lengthwise
2 teaspoons chillie powder
1 teaspoon chopped ginger
1 teaspoon chopped garlic
Salt to taste
2 tablespoons oil
½ cup thick tamarind juice

Heat oil in a pressure cooker and sauté the onions lightly. Add the trotters and all the other ingredients (except the tamarind Juice) and mix well. Fry for a few minutes. Add sufficient water and pressure cook on medium heat for about 15 minutes. Open the pressure cooker and add the thick tamarind juice and mix well. Continue cooking on low heat till the gravy is thick and dark brown. Serve with Chapattis, Hoppers or Dosas.

67. Spicy Trotters Curry

Serves 6   *Preparation Time 1 hour*

Ingredients

8 Trotters (Mutton or Lamb) preferably the front ones
1 teaspoon ginger garlic paste
2 pieces cinnamon (about ½ inch each)
3 cloves
2 large tomatoes chopped
2 teaspoons chillie powder
2 large onions chopped
1 teaspoon coriander powder
½ teaspoon turmeric powder
1 teaspoon cumin powder
2 tablespoons vinegar
3 tablespoons oil
Salt to taste
2 tablespoons coriander leaves chopped.

Heat oil in a pressure cooker and lightly sauté the onions, cinnamon and cloves. Add the trotters, ginger garlic paste, turmeric powder, chillie powder, tomato, coriander powder, cumin powder, vinegar and salt and mix well. Add sufficient water and pressure cook first on high heat then on low heat for half an hour or till the trotters are well cooked. Garnish with chopped coriander leaves. Serve hot with rice or bread or even dosas or hoppers.

68. Ox Tail Vindaloo

Serves 6   *Preparation time 45 minutes*

Ingredients

1 kg oxtail cut into medium pieces
3 onions chopped
3 big tomatoes pureed
1 teaspoon cumin powder
1 teaspoon turmeric powder
3 teaspoons chillie powder
1 teaspoon pepper powder
1 piece cinnamon
2 teaspoons garlic paste
3 tablespoons vinegar
3 tablespoons oil
Salt to taste

Pressure cook the oxtail till soft with sufficient water. Heat oil and fry the cinnamon and onions till golden brown. Add the garlic paste and sauté for some time. Add the chillie powder, cumin powder, turmeric powder, pepper powder and fry well with a little vinegar. Add the tomato puree and continue frying till the oil separates from the mixture. Add the remaining vinegar and the cooked oxtail together with the remaining soup and cook till the gravy is thick. Serve hot with rice or bread or even hoppers.

69. Ox Tail Puli Sauce
(Ox Tail in a Tangy Tamarind Base)

This version of Ox tail is finger licking good!!

Serves 6   Preparation time 45 minutes

Ingredients

1 Ox tail chopped into medium size pieces
2 big onions sliced
1 teaspoon coriander powder
4 green chillies slit lengthwise
2 teaspoons chillie powder
1 teaspoon chopped ginger
1 teaspoon chopped garlic
Salt to taste
2 tablespoons oil
½ cup thick tamarind juice

Heat oil in a pressure cooker and sauté the onions lightly. Add the pieces of the Ox tail and all the other ingredients (except the tamarind Juice) and mix well. Fry for a few minutes. Add sufficient water and pressure cook on medium heat for about 15 minutes. Open the pressure cooker and now add the thick tamarind juice and mix well. Continue cooking on low heat till the gravy is thick and dark brown. Serve with Chapattis, Hoppers or Dosas.

70. Lamb / Sheep Head Curry

Serves 6   Preparation Time 45 minutes

Ingredients

1 goat / sheep's head skinned and cut into medium pieces
3 tablespoon's oil

2 large onions chopped finely
2 green chilies slit lengthwise
2 tablespoons ginger garlic paste
½ teaspoon turmeric powder
2 teaspoons chillie powder
2 teaspoons cumin powder
2 teaspoons coriander powder
1 teaspoon mustard powder
Salt to taste
2 teaspoons chopped garlic

Wash the pieces of goat / sheep's head well. Boil with a little water in a suitable pan or pressure cooker till cooked. In another vessel, sauté the onions, green chilies and the ginger garlic paste for some time. Add the chillie powder, cumin powder, coriander powder, turmeric powder, mustard powder and fry for some time with a little water. Add the cooked sheep's head pieces along with the soup, chopped garlic and salt and simmer till the gravy is thick. Garnish with chopped coriander if deserved.

---

71. Curried Brain

Serves 6   *Preparation Time approx 1 hour*

Ingredients

3 Sheep brains or 1 Ox brain
2 Onions chopped finely
2 tablespoons oil
2 Tomatoes chopped
1 teaspoon chopped garlic
Salt to taste
2 teaspoons chillie powder
½ teaspoon turmeric powder
1 teaspoon coriander leaves chopped for garnishing

Clean and wash the brains well. Steam them in some hot water with a pinch of salt for about 5 minutes. Drain and keep aside. When cold, slice them into 10 or 12 pieces.

Heat the oil in a suitable pan and sauté the chopped garlic and onions till golden brown. Add all the other ingredients and stir fry for about 3 minutes. Add the steamed brain prices and gently mix so that all the pieces are covered with the gravy. Simmer for about 3 more minutes. Garnish with chopped Coriander leaves. Serve with bread or rice.

72. Brain And Onion Leeks (Spring Onions) Curry

Serves 6   Preparation Time approx 1 hour

Ingredients

4 sheep Brains or 1 Ox brain cut into medium size pieces
1 cup fresh Spring Onions / Onions Leeks (wash and cut into suitable sizes depending on choice)
1 teaspoon ginger and garlic paste
1 teaspoon spice powder or garam masala powder
2 teaspoons chillie powder
3 onions sliced
2 tomatoes chopped
Salt to taste
3 green chillies
½ teaspoon turmeric powder
½ teaspoon coriander powder
2 tablespoons oil

Heat oil in a pan and fry the onions well. Add the green chillies, ginger and garlic paste and sauté lightly. Add the tomato, chillie powder, spice powder, turmeric powder and coriander powder and fry for some time. Add the chopped spring onions and mix well. Continue frying for some time till the oil separates from the mixture and the spring onions are just cooked. Add the brain and mix gently. Cover and cook on low heat for 5 more minutes. Serve with rice, bread or chapattis.

---

73. Brain Pepper Fry

Serves 6   *Preparation Time 30 minutes*

Ingredients

4 Sheep Brains or 1 calf Brain
2 onions sliced finely
Salt to taste
2 teaspoons pepper powder
2 table spoons oil

Wash the Brain well and remove the top skin. Fry the onions till golden brown. Add the Brain and sauté for some time. Sprinkle the salt and Pepper powder on the brain and mix carefully. Cover and steam cook for about 6 minutes till the brain is cooked.

Garnish with slit green chilies

Note: A teaspoon of chillie powder can be used instead of pepper powder for a variation in taste.

---

74. Spicy Brain Fry

Serves 6   *Preparation Time approx 1 hour*

Ingredients

4 Sheep brains or 1 Ox Brain
2 Onions chopped finely
2 tablespoons oil
2 Tomatoes chopped
1 teaspoon chopped garlic

Salt to taste
2 teaspoons chillie powder
½ teaspoon turmeric powder
1 teaspoon coriander leaves chopped for garnishing

Clean and wash the brains well. Steam them in some hot water with a pinch of salt for about 5 minutes. Drain and keep aside. When cold, slice them into 10 or 12 pieces.

Heat the oil in a suitable pan and sauté the chopped garlic and onions till golden brown. Add all the other ingredients and stir fry for about 5 minutes. Add the steamed brain pieces and mix gently so that all the pieces are covered with the gravy. Simmer for about 3 more minutes. Garnish with chopped Coriander leaves. Serve with bread or rice.

75. Brain Cutlets

Serves 6   Preparation Time 45 minutes

Ingredients

4 Sheep's brains or 1 calf brain
1 teaspoon pepper powder
½ teaspoon salt
2 tablespoons breadcrumbs
1 teaspoon chopped mint or ½ teaspoon dry mint
2 slices bread soaked in water and squeezed dry
1 egg (The white and the yolk to be beaten separately)
2 tablespoons oil

Wash the Brains well and remove the skin. Boil with a little water in a pan for 3 minutes. Drain and keep aside to cool. When quite cold, break into small pieces and mix with the salt, pepper, mint, soaked bread and the egg yolk. Divide and shape into cutlets. Dip each cutlet in the egg whites and coat with breadcrumbs on both sides. Heat the oil on a flat pan and shallow fry the cutlets on low heat till brown on both sides.

---

76. Savoury Brain Fritters

Serves 6   Preparation time 1 hour

Ingredients

3 Sheep Brains or ½ kg Beef Brain
2 teaspoons pepper powder
4 tablespoons flour (Maida)
2 green chillies chopped finely
1 egg beaten
Salt to taste
Oil for frying

Wash the Brains well and remove the veins etc. Cut them into 1" pieces. Make a batter with the beaten egg, flour, salt, pepper powder, chillies and a little water. Mix with the pieces of brain. Heat oil in a pan and drop in the batter covered brain and deep fry till golden brown. Serve hot.

For a difference in taste, use Besan flour instead of Maida and finely chopped green chillies, green coriander and onions may be added to the batter.

---

77. Simple Anglo-Indian Beef Roast

Serves 6   Preparation time 1 hour

Ingredients

2 kg Beef from the "Round Portion" or "Top Rump part"
2 large onions cut into quarters
2 teaspoons pepper powder

Salt to taste
3 tablespoons oil
3 large potatoes pealed

Wash the meat and rub the salt and pepper well into it. Heat the oil in a big pan or a pressure cooker, and add the meat to it. Cook on high heat for a few minutes, turning the meat on all sides till it changes colour. Add the onions, potatoes and sufficient water and cook on low heat till the meat is tender. Continue to simmer on low heat till the meat is nicely brown all over and the potatoes too are nicely roasted. Serve hot or cold with bread. (If cooking in a pressure cooker switch off after 20 minutes).

The same recipe can be used for making Mutton or Lamb Roast as well.

---

78. Beef Pot Roast

Serves 6   *Preparation time 11/2 hour*

Ingredients

2 kg Beef from the "Top Rump part" (one chunk)
3 large onions cut into quarters
3 teaspoons pepper powder
Salt to taste
3 dried red chillies or 1 teaspoon Paprika
2 pieces of cinnamon (about one inch size)
2 teaspoons Tomato sauce
2 teaspoons vinegar
3 tablespoons oil
3 large potatoes pealed
2 tablespoons butter or ghee

Marinate the chunk of beef with salt and pepper for about one hour. Heat the oil in a big Pan or pressure cooker and add the chunk of meat. Fry on high heat for about 3 minutes, turning the meat on all sides till it changes colour. Add the onions, tomato sauce, vinegar, dry chillies, cinnamon, potatoes and sufficient water and simmer till the meat is tender. Strain away any excess soup and keep aside.

Add 2 tablespoons of butter or ghee and continue to simmer on low heat till the meat is nicely brown all over and the potatoes too are nicely roasted. Slice the meat and arrange on a serving platter.

Pour the remaining soup back into the pan and mix in 2 tablespoons of flour. Cook till the gravy thickens, stirring all the time. Spoon this gravy on top of the slices of roast and serve the remaining gravy on the side along with the Roast potatoes.

(Alternatively the meat could be cooked in a pressure cooker till soft and then browned in a pan).

---

79. Roast Leg Of Lamb

Serves 6   Preparation time 1 hour

Ingredients

1 whole leg of mutton /Lamb
3 large potatoes
2 tablespoons vinegar
2 teaspoons pepper
Salt to taste

Wash the lamb / mutton leg and make deep cuts on it. Rub it well all over with the salt, pepper and vinegar. Place it in a big oven proof dish or pressure cooker and fry for some time till slightly brown. Add the potatoes and sufficient water and cook till the meat is tender. Continue roasting till the meat is nice and brown and the potatoes too are roasted well. Serve hot or cold with bread steaned vegetables.

80. Ox Tongue Roast

Serves 6   *Preparation time 1 hour*

Ingredients

1 large Ox tongue
1 big onion sliced
4 Red chilies broken into bits
1 teaspoon peppercorns
2 cloves and 2 pieces of cinnamon
2 tablespoons oil
Salt to taste

Wash the tongue well and then pressure cook it with 2 cups of water and a little salt till tender letting some soup remain. Open the pressure cooker and remove the boiled tongue. Let it cool for some time. When a little cold remove the white skin from the tongue and put it back into the open cooker and add the oil, onion, red chilies pepper corns, cloves and cinnamon and a little more salt. Mix well. Simmer on low heat till all the soup dries up and the tongue is nicely brown all over. Cut into slices and arrange on a plate along with the residue. Serve hot or cold with mash potatoes and bread. You can make delicious sandwiches with tongue roast as filling.

C. Pork

1. Pork Vindaloo

Serves 6   Preparation Time 45 minutes

Ingredients

1 kg pork cut into medium pieces
3 big onions sliced finely
1 tablespoon cumin powder
½ teaspoon turmeric powder
1 teaspoon mustard powder
3 teaspoons chillie powder
2 teaspoons pepper powder
3 teaspoons garlic paste
1 cup vinegar
3 tablespoons oil
1 sprig curry leaves
Salt to taste

Marinate the pork for about one hour with the salt, vinegar, chillie powder, cumin powder pepper powder, mustard powder, turmeric powder and garlic paste. Heat oil in a pressure cooker and fry the curry leaves and onions till golden brown. Add the marinated pork and keep frying for some time. Now add more water and pressure cook till the meat is well cooked. Serve hot with rice or bread.

2. Country Captain Pork

Serves 6   *Preparation Time 30 minutes*

Ingredients

1 kg pork cut into medium size pieces
3 large onions sliced finely
2 teaspoons chillie powder
1 teaspoon turmeric powder
2 tablespoons oil
Salt to taste
2 tablespoons garlic paste
2 sticks cinnamon
4 cloves
2 cardamoms
2 tablespoons vinegar

Wash the pork and boil with a little salt and 1 cup water till tender. Heat oil in a pan and fry the onions lightly. Add the garlic paste and sauté for about 5 minutes on medium heat. Add the chillie powder, turmeric powder, cinnamon, cloves, cardamom, vinegar and salt. Now add the cooked pork along with the soup and simmer for about 10 minutes till the gravy is thick. Serve with bread or rice.

3. Spicy Pork Curry

Serves 6   *Preparation Time 45 minutes*

Ingredients

1 kg pork with the fat and lard cut into medium pieces
3 big onions sliced finely
3 big tomatoes pureed
1 tablespoon cumin powder
2 teaspoons coriander powder

½ teaspoon turmeric powder
1 teaspoon mustard seeds
3 teaspoons chillie powder
8 or 10 curry leaves
3 tablespoons ginger garlic paste
3 tablespoons oil
Salt to taste

Make a powder of 3 cardamoms, 3 cloves, 2 sticks cinnamon and 2 teaspoons aniseeds or saunf.

Wash the pork and set aside Heat oil in a pressure cooker and add the mustard seeds. When they begin to crackle add the curry leaves and onions and fry till golden brown. Now add the chillie powder, cumin powder, turmeric powder, coriander powder, powdered spices and ginger garlic paste and fry for some time. Add the pork, salt and the tomato puree and keep frying for some time. Add sufficient water and pressure cook for about 20 minutes on high heat till the pork is cooked. Serve hot with rice or bread.

---

4. Old Madras Pork Curry

Serves 6   Preparation Time 45 minutes

Ingredients

½ kg Pork cut into medium pieces without lard
2 tomatoes chopped
2 large onions sliced finely
3 green chilies sliced lengthwise
2 teaspoons ginger garlic paste
3 tablespoons oil
2 teaspoons chillie Powder
½ teaspoons turmeric Powder
Salt to taste
2 potatoes boiled and peeled

Wash the pork and cook it together with the tomato, turmeric and salt in sufficient water till tender. Let a little soup remain. Add the chillie powder, green chilies, sliced onions, ginger and garlic paste and mix well. Cook on low heat till the soup dries up. Add the oil and keep on frying on low heat till the meat turns brown. Serve with bread or rice. Add boiled potatoes and mix well before taking down.

5. Pork With Dill Leaves and Potatoes

Serves 6   *Preparation Time 45 minutes*

Ingredients

1 kg Pork with less fat cut into medium pieces
1 teaspoon ginger paste
1 teaspoon garlic paste
½ teaspoon turmeric Powder
2 teaspoon chillie Powder
2 green chillies sliced lengthwise
3 onions sliced finely
1 cup chopped Dill leaves
Salt to taste
3 Potatoes peeled and cut into quarters
3 tablespoons oil

Heat oil in a pan and fry the onions till golden brown. Add the ginger and garlic paste and sauté for a few more minutes. Add the pork, chillie powder, turmeric powder, green chillies and Dill leaves and mix well. Stir fry for a few minutes till the pork pieces become firm and the leaves shrivel up. Add the potatoes, salt and sufficient water and simmer on low heat till the pork and potatoes are tender.

6. Devilled Pork

Serves 6   Preparation Time 45 minutes

Ingredients

1 kg Pork (less fat) cut into medium size pieces
2 tablespoons vinegar
1 tablespoon Worcester sauce or Soya Sauce
2 tablespoons Tomato sauce
3 tablespoons oil
3 large onions sliced
2 tablespoons chopped garlic
2 tablespoons chopped ginger
8 to 10 Curry Leaves
1 tablespoon sugar
1 teaspoon fenugreek seeds powdered (Methi)
1 teaspoon mustard powder or paste
2 pieces cinnamon
3 cloves
3 teaspoons chillie powder
1 teaspoon turmeric powder
Salt to taste
2 tablespoons oil

Marinate the pork with the Vinegar, Worcester / Soya Sauce, Tomato Sauce, sugar and salt for about 1 hour. Heat oil in a pressure Cooker or pan and sauté the onions, curry leaves, chopped ginger, chopped garlic, cinnamon and cloves till light brown. Add the marinated pork, chillie powder, turmeric powder, fenugreek powder, mustard and mix well. Simmer for a few minutes till the meat becomes firm. Add sufficient water and pressure cook for about 15 to 20 minutes till the pork is cooked. Open the pressure cooker and simmer till the gravy is thick. Serve with Rice, Bread or Chappatis.

7. Spicy Pork Liver Fry

Serves 6   Preparation time 1 hour

Ingredients

½ kg pork liver cut into medium size pieces
4 onions sliced finely
4 green chillies
3 teaspoons pepper powder
2 teaspoons cumin powder
½ teaspoon turmeric powder
1 teaspoon all spice powder
1 tablespoon ginger garlic paste
1 tablespoon red chillie powder
1 tablespoon vinegar
2 tablespoons oil
Salt to taste

Wash the liver pieces and cook it in sufficient water till soft with a little salt. Remove from the heat and strain away the soup. Fry these pieces lightly in a little oil and keep aside. Add a little more oil to the pan, then fry the sliced onions, and green chillies for a few minutes. Add the ginger garlic paste and sauté for some time. Next add all the other ingredients and the left over soup and mix well. Simmer on low heat for 5 minutes. Add the fried liver pieces, vinegar and salt to taste and simmer on low heat till the gravy is quite thick. Serve with bread or rice.

8. Pork Bafat

Serves 6   Preparation Time 45 minutes

Ingredients

1 kg pork cut into medium size pieces (with the lard and fat)
3 onions chopped

2 green chillies slit lengthwise
2 teaspoons chopped garlic
1 teaspoon chopped ginger
2 pieces cinnamon (one inch size)
4 cloves
2 bay leaves
2 teaspoons chillie powder
1 teaspoon coriander powder
I teaspoon cumin powder
1 teaspoon all spice powder or garam masala powder
2 tablespoons vinegar
Salt to taste

Marinate the pork with all the above ingredients for one hour. Transfer to a suitable pan and simmer on low heat till the pork is cooked and gravy is quite thick. (Add a little water while cooking if more gravy is required) For an extra Tangy taste, add a little tamarind or lime juice while cooking. Serve hot with bread, rice or dosas.

Note: A teaspoon of Readymade Bafat Powder could also be used to add to the taste.

9. Spicy Pork Fry

Serves 6   *Preparation Time 1 hour*

Ingredients

1 kg tender pork (less fat) cut into cubes
3 onions sliced finely
8 or 9 curry leaves
2 teaspoons ginger and garlic paste
½ teaspoon turmeric powder
3 teaspoons chillie powder
1 teaspoon cumin powder
2 cloves

2 small pieces of cinnamon
2 tablespoons vinegar
Salt to taste

Boil the pork with a little salt and a pinch of turmeric in sufficient water till tender. Strain the soup and keep aside. Heat oil in a pan and sauté the onions, cinnamon, cloves and curry leaves till slightly brown. Add the ginger and garlic paste, chillie powder, cumin powder, turmeric powder and vinegar and fry for a few minutes. Add the cooked pork and mix well. Add the remaining soup and simmer till almost dry.

---

10. Pork Pepper Fry

Serves 6   *Preparation Time 1 hour*

Ingredients

1 kg tender pork cut into cubes
2 green chillies sliced
3 onions sliced finely
½ teaspoon turmeric powder
3 teaspoons pepper powder
Salt to taste

Cook the pork with a little salt and a pinch of turmeric in sufficient water till tender. Strain the soup and keep aside. Heat oil in a pan and sauté the onions and green chillies till slightly brown. Add the cooked pork, pepper powder, turmeric powder and salt and fry for a few minutes. Add the left over soup / stock and mix well. Simmer on low heat till almost dry and dark in colour.

11. Pork Chillie Fry

Serves 6   *Preparation Time 45 minutes*

Ingredients:

1 kg Pork without the lard cut into small pieces
3 large onions sliced finely
8 peppercorns
1 teaspoon chopped ginger
1 teaspoon chopped garlic
6 or 8 green chillies sliced lengthwise (reduce the chillies if too pungent)
Salt to taste
3 tablespoons oil

Boil the Pork with a little salt and the peppercorns in sufficient water till tender. Drain the left over soup and keep aside. Heat oil in a pan and fry the onions, slit green chillies, ginger and garlic till light brown. Add the boiled pork and a little more salt if necessary and cook on low heat till almost dry. Serve with rice or bread.

12. Fried Pork Loin

Serves 6   *Preparation Time 45 minutes*

Ingredients

1 kg boneless Pork Loin cut into long thin slices
½ cup flour or maida
Salt to taste
1 tablespoon butter
2 tablespoons oil
2 tablespoons vinegar
2 teaspoons pepper powder

Marinate the Pork strips with the vinegar, flour, salt, pepper and butter and set aside for about one hour. Heat oil in a pan and add the marinated pork strips. Simmer on low heat, turning the strips over occasionally till tender and well browned all over. Add some water while cooking if required. Serve as a side dish with other curries and rice.

13. Pepper Pork Chops

Serves 6   *Preparation Time 45 minutes*

Ingredients

½ kg good pork chops (Flatten them)
3 potatoes (Boiled, pealed and cut in half lengthwise)
4 big onions sliced
2 green chilies slit lengthwise
2 teaspoons pepper powder
Salt to taste
3 tablespoons oil

Pressure cook the pork chops with a little water till tender letting some soup remain. Open the pressure cooker and add the onions, green chilies, salt, pepper powder and oil and mix well. Keep cooking on low heat till the soup dries up and the onions and pork are nicely browned. Just before turning off the heat add the boiled potatoes and mix well. Serve hot with bread or rice as a side dish.

14. Pork Chops In Gravy

Serves 6   *Preparation Time 1 hour*

Ingredients

½ kg good pork chops
2 teaspoons ginger garlic paste
2 tablespoons vinegar
2 large onions sliced finely
2 or 3 green chilies sliced lengthwise
2 tablespoons oil
3 teaspoons chillie powder
1 teaspoon spice powder or garam masala
1 teaspoon pepper powder
Salt to taste

Wash the chops and marinate them with the ginger garlic paste, pepper powder, spice powder, vinegar, chillie powder and salt for about one hour. Heat oil in a large pan and sauté the onions, and green chilies for a few minutes. Add the marinated chops and mix well. Simmer for a few minutes. Add sufficient water and cook till the chops are done and the gravy is thick. Garnish with onion rings.

15. Savoury Pork Chops

Serves 6   *Preparation Time 30 minutes*

Ingredients

1 kg pork chops flattened
3 large onions sliced finely
2 teaspoons chillie powder
1 teaspoon turmeric powder
2 tablespoons oil
Salt to taste

2 tablespoons garlic paste
2 sticks cinnamon
4 cloves
2 cardamoms
1 teaspoon cumin powder
2 red chillies broken into bits
2 tablespoons vinegar

Boil the Pork Chops in a little water till tender. Strain the stock
and keep aside. Heat oil in a pan and fry the onions, red chillies,
cinnamon, cloves and cardamom lightly. Add the garlic paste
and sauté for about 5 minutes on medium heat. Add the chillie
powder, cumin powder, turmeric powder, salt and the pork
along with the vinegar and cook on medium heat till the chops
turn brown and semi dry. Serve with bread or rice.

16. Spicy Pork Chops

Serves 6   *Preparation Time 45 minutes*

Ingredients

1 kg Pork Chops
4 green chilies ground to a paste
2 teaspoons lime juice
1 teaspoon mustard powder
3 tablespoons Worcestershire / Soya sauce
2 teaspoons chillie powder
1 teaspoon Coriander powder
Salt to taste
2 tablespoons oil
1 teaspoon peppercorns
3 onions sliced finely
2 tablespoons vinegar
2 one inch pieces of cinnamon
3 cloves
3 Potatoes boiled and cut into halves

Marinate the chops with all the above ingredients (except the potatoes) for about one hour. Transfer to a suitable pan and cook on high heat for about 3 minutes stirring occasionally. Add 2 cups water and simmer on low heat till the chops are tender and the gravy is thick. Add the Potatoes and mix once. Serve with Rice or bread.

17. Pork Spare Ribs

Serves 6   *Preparation Time 45 minutes*

Ingredients

1 kg Pork Spare Ribs
2 teaspoons coriander powder
1 teaspoon cumin powder
2 teaspoon finely chopped garlic
2 tablespoons oil
Salt to taste
2 teaspoons chillie Powder
2 teaspoons tomato sauce / ketchup
2 tablespoons vinegar
3 onions finely chopped

Marinate the Pork Spare Ribs with the coriander powder, cumin powder, chillie powder, vinegar, tomato sauce / ketchup and salt for one hour. Heat oil in a pan and sauté the onions and chopped garlic till golden brown. Add the marinated Pork Spare Ribs and mix well. Add sufficient water and cook till tender. Serve with rice or Bread.

18. Pepper Pork Spare Ribs

Serves 6   *Preparation Time 45 minutes*

Ingredients

1 kg Pork Spare Ribs
2 teaspoons Coriander Powder
2 teaspoon finely chopped garlic
2 tablespoons oil
Salt to taste
2 teaspoons ground pepper powder
3 onions finely chopped

Marinate the Pork Spare Ribs with the coriander, pepper powder, and salt for one hour. Heat oil in a pan and sauté the onions and chopped garlic till golden brown. Add the marinated Pork Spare Ribs and mix well. Add sufficient water and cook till tender. Serve with rice or Bread.

19. Curried Pork Trotters

Serves 6   *Preparation Time 1 hour*

Ingredients

8 pig Trotters preferably the front ones
2 large tomatoes pureed
3 teaspoons chillie powder
2 large onions chopped
1 teaspoon coriander powder
1 teaspoon all spice powder or garam masala powder
3 tablespoons oil
Salt to taste

A small bunch of coriander leaves chopped.

Wash the trotters well and cook it with sufficient water and a little salt in a pressure cooker till soft.

Heat oil in a pan and lightly sauté the onions. Add the cooked trotters, all spice powder, chillie powder, coriander powder, tomato puree, salt and mix well. Cook first on high heat then on low heat for for about 15 minutes. Garnish with chopped coriander leaves. Serve hot with rice or bread or even dosas or hoppers.

20. Pepper Pork Mince Fry

Serves 6   Preparation Time 45 minutes

Ingredients

½ kg Pork Mince
2 big onions chopped
½ teaspoon turmeric powder
1 teaspoon chopped garlic
2 green chilies chopped finely
2 tablespoons oil
Salt to taste
2 teaspoons pepper powder
2 Potatoes boiled and chopped into small pieces

Heat oil in a pan and fry the chopped garlic and onions till golden brown. Add the green chilies, turmeric powder, pepper powder and sauté for 2 minutes. Add the mince and salt and a little water mix well. Cook on low heat for about ½ an hour till the mince is cooked and all the water evaporates. Add the Potatoes and mix well. Simmer on low heat for 3 more minutes. Serve hot with bread or chapattis.

21. Home-Made Pork Pepper Sausages

Makes around 15 sausages

Preparation time 1 hour

Ingredients

1 kg Ground pork (add a little quantity of small finely cut pieces of Fat to the mince)
2 pieces cinnamon about 1 inch each
4 cloves
1/2 teaspoon nutmeg powder
Salt to taste
2 teaspoons pepper corns
1 teaspoon garlic paste
2 tablespoon chopped coriander leaves (optional)
3 tablespoons bread crumbs
Sufficient quantity of casing for stuffing the sausages

Roughly powder the cinnamon, cloves and pepper. Mix all the ingredients together well and stuff into the casing. Grill or Fry when required. These sausages should be kept in the refrigerator and used up within 2 weeks as no preservatives have been used.

22. Pork Sausage Curry

Serves 6   Preparation Time 45 minutes

Ingredients

500 grams pork pepper sausages
2 big tomatoes chopped
2 large onions sliced finely
2 green chilies sliced lengthwise
1 teaspoon ginger garlic paste

1 teaspoon chopped garlic
2 tablespoons oil
1 teaspoon chillie powder
½ teaspoon turmeric powder
½ teaspoon coriander powder
½ teaspoon cumin powder
Salt to taste

Heat oil in a pan and add the sausages and a little water. Cook on low heat till the water evaporates and the sausages turn golden brown. Remove from heat and slice the sausages into halves.

In the same oil add the onions, chopped garlic and green chillies and fry till golden brown. Add the ginger garlic paste and fry for 2 or 3 minutes. Now add the tomatoes, turmeric, chillie powder, coriander powder, cumin powder and salt and fry till the tomatoes turn pulpy. Add 1 cup of water and bring to boil. Add the sliced sausages and cook on low heat till the gravy becomes thick. Serve with bread or rice.

---

23. Simple Pork Roast

Serves 6   Preparation time 1 hour

Ingredients

1 whole chunk of pork weighing around 2 kgs
3 large potatoes peeled
2 tablespoons vinegar
2 teaspoons pepper
Salt to taste

Wash the chunk of pork and make deep cuts on it. Rub it well all over with the salt, pepper and vinegar. Place it in a big pan or pressure cooker and fry for some time till slightly brown on all sides. Add the potatoes and sufficient water and cook till the meat is tender. Continue roasting till the meat is nice and brown and the potatoes too are roasted well. Serve hot or cold with bread.

---

24. Pork Pot Roast

Serves 6   *Preparation time 1 hour*

Ingredients

1 chunk of pork weighing around 2 kgs with fat and lard
3 potatoes peeled
3 whole red chillies
1 teaspoon pepper corns
3 cloves
3 cardamoms,
1 Bay leaf
Salt to taste

Wash the pork and rub well with the salt and a pinch of pepper. Place in a pressure cooker together with the red chillies, peppercorns, spices, bay leaf and a little water and pressure – cook for 15 minutes. Open the pressure cooker and add the whole potatoes. Simmer on low heat turning the meat around till nicely browned on all sides.

Alternately, the meat can be roasted with all the above ingredients in an oven for 2 hours or till the meat is soft and brown.

25. Home-Made Salted Pork

Serves 6

Ingredients

2 kg Chunk of Boneless Pork (preferably from the Belly Portion) with the skin
1 teaspoon saltpetre or lime salt
8 teaspoons table salt or powdered salt
3 teaspoons sugar
2 tablespoons vinegar

Mix the saltpetre / lime salt, table salt, sugar and vinegar together. Rub this mixture on the pork and prick all over with a fork. Keep in the fridge for 4 or 5 days turning it over and rubbing it well several times a day. On the 6th day boil in a suitable vessel with the residue and a little water for about one hour or pressure cook for 35 minutes on low heat. Cool and store and use whenever required.

D. Fish and Seafood

---

1. Fish Vindaloo

Serves 6   *Preparation Time 45 minutes*

Ingredients

1 kg good fleshy fish cut into slices
2 medium sized onions chopped
2 teaspoons chillie powder
2 teaspoons cumin powder
2 teaspoons garlic paste
2 tablespoons vinegar
Salt to taste
1 sprig curry leaves (optional)
2 tomatoes pureed or chopped finely
2 tablespoons oil

Wash the fish well and lightly fry in a little oil till the pieces become firm. Keep aside. Heat oil in a pan and add the curry leaves and onions and fry till light brown. Add the garlic paste and sauté for a while. Add the chillie powder, cumin powder, tomato puree and salt and fry for some time. Add the fish and the vinegar and mix well. Add a just a little more water and cook till the gravy is slightly thick.

2. Tangy Fish Curry

(Fish cooked in Tamarind Sauce)

Serves 6   Preparation Time 45 minutes

Ingredients

1 kg good fleshy fish cut into slices
½ cup thick tamarind juice extracted from a lime size ball of
tamarind
2 big onions chopped finely
2 tablespoons ginger garlic paste
3 teaspoons chillie powder
1 teaspoon cumin powder
2 teaspoons coriander powder
½ teaspoon turmeric powder
Salt to taste
3 tablespoons oil

Wash the fish well and fry it lightly to make it firm. Heat the oil
in a shallow vessel and fry the onions till golden brown. Add
the ginger garlic paste, chillie powder, cumin powder, coriander
powder, turmeric powder and a little water and fry well for
some time. Add the salt, tamarind juice and a little more water
and bring to boil. Add the fish and cook for about 6 to 7 minutes
till the fish is cooked. Garnish with chopped coriander leaves
and slit green chilies.

3. Fish Moley

(Fish Stew cooked with green chillies and coconut milk)

Serves 6   Preparation Time 45 minutes

Ingredients

1 kg good fleshy fish sliced thickly or in fillets
3 big onions sliced finely
4 to 5 green chilies sliced lengthwise
1 teaspoon chopped garlic
1 teaspoon chopped ginger
1cup thick coconut milk
1 tomato chopped into fairly big pieces
6 or 7 curry leaves
1 teaspoon ground pepper powder
½ teaspoon chillie powder
½ teaspoon turmeric powder
1 teaspoon coriander powder
½ teaspoon mustard seeds
1 tablespoon lime juice or vinegar
3 tablespoons oil
Salt to taste

Wash the fish well and rub all over with the turmeric powder and a little salt. Heat oil in a pan and lightly fry the fish till golden. Remove and keep aside.

In the same pan add a little more oil if required and add the mustard seeds. When they begin to crackle add the onions, garlic and ginger and sauté till the onions turn golden brown. Add the chopped tomato and curry leaves and fry for a minute. Add the salt, pepper powder, slit green chillies, chillie powder, coriander powder and lime juice / vinegar and mix well. Add the coconut milk and a little water and mix well. Simmer for a few minutes till the gravy thickens. Slowly add the fried fish to this gravy. Shake the pan so that all the pieces of fish get covered well. Cook on medium heat for 2 minutes till the fish absorbs the flavours and the gravy thickens.

Serve with rice or hoppers.

---

4. Fish In Tomato Gravy

Serves 6   *Preparation Time 20 minutes*

Ingredients

½ kg of any fleshy fish cut into thick pieces
3 tablespoons oil
2 teaspoons ginger garlic paste
3 tomatoes pureed
2 teaspoons chillie powder
1 teaspoon cumin powder
Salt to taste
¼ teaspoon turmeric powder
1 tablespoon vinegar
3 onions sliced finely

Wash the fish and keep aside. Heat oil in a pan and sauté the onions for a few minutes. Add the ginger garlic paste, chillie powder, cumin powder, turmeric powder and salt and fry for a few minutes. Add the tomato puree and vinegar and mix well. Fry for a few minutes. Add ½ cup of water and bring to boil. Drop in the fish pieces and mix well. Simmer on low heat till the fish is cooked. Serve with bread or chapattis.

5. Pomfret Curry

Serves 6   *Preparation Time 45 minutes*

Ingredients

1 kg good fleshy pomfrets sliced thickly
3 big onions sliced finely
2 green chilies sliced lengthwise
1 tablespoon ginger garlic paste
3 tablespoons ground coconut paste or coconut milk
½ teaspoon turmeric powder
3 tablespoons oil
Salt to taste
1cup thick tamarind juice or ½ cup lime juice
3 teaspoons chillie powder
1 teaspoon cumin powder
1 teaspoon coriander powder
2 sprigs curry leaves

Heat oil in a pan and add the curry leaves and onions and sauté for a few minutes. Add the ginger garlic paste, turmeric powder, chillie powder, cumin powder, coriander powder and coconut and fry for 2 or 3 minutes. Add the tamarind juice, salt and slit green chillies and bring to boil. Add the fish and a little more water if more gravy is required. Cook on low heat for about 5 minutes till the fish is cooked. Pour a tablespoon of oil on top then remove from heat. (Care should be taken not to over cook the fish or else it will break up.) Serve with rice or bread.

6. Green Masala Pomfret Curry

Serves 6   Preparation Time 45 minutes

Ingredients

3 medium size pomfrets cut into medium pieces
2 teaspoons ginger garlic paste
4 green chillies
4 tablespoons coriander leaves
1 teaspoon cumin powder
2 cloves
2 cardamom
2 pieces of cinnamon
½ teaspoon turmeric powder
Salt to taste
3 tablespoons oil
2 onions sliced finely
½ cup coconut paste
2 teaspoons chopped mint

Grind the green chilies, coriander leaves, mint leaves, coconut, cinnamon, cloves, cardamom and cumin to a smooth paste in a blender. Heat oil in a pan and fry the onions till golden brown. Add the ginger garlic paste, turmeric powder and fry for some time. Now add the ground masala and salt and mix well. Keep frying on low heat till the oil separates from the masala. Add the pomfret and sufficient water to cover the fish and cook for 5 to 6 minutes. Serve hot.

7. King Fish / Seer Fish And Green Mango Curry

Serves 6   Preparation Time 45 minutes

Ingredients

½ Kg King Fish / Seer Fish slices / Spanish Blue Mackerel
1 teaspoon ginger garlic paste
1 teaspoon coriander powder
1 teaspoon cumin powder
2 teaspoons chillie powder
½ teaspoon turmeric powder
Salt to taste
3 tablespoons oil
2 green mangoes peeled and cut into medium size pieces
2 onions sliced finely
½ cup coconut paste
2 green chilies
3 tablespoons coriander leaves to garnish

Cook the green mango pieces with the green chillies and a pinch of turmeric in a little water till soft.

Heat oil in a pan and fry the onions till golden brown. Add the ginger garlic paste and sauté for a few minutes. Add the turmeric powder, chillie powder, cumin powder, coriander powder, coconut paste and salt and mix well. Keep frying on low heat till the oil separates from the mixture. Add the fish and the cooked mango pieces and a little water and cook for 5 to 6 minutes till the fish is done. Garnish with the chopped coriander leaves. Serve hot with rice.

8. King Fish / Seer Fish In Coconut Gravy

(King fish is also known as Sea Mullet / Round head / Sea Mink etc)

Serves 6   *Preparation Time 45 minutes*

Ingredients

1 kg good King Fish / Seer Fish cut into slices
2 big onions chopped finely
2 teaspoons garlic ginger paste
1 cup thick coconut milk
3 teaspoons chillie powder
1 teaspoon cumin powder
2 teaspoons coriander powder
½ teaspoon turmeric powder
A few Curry Leaves
Salt to taste
3 tablespoons oil (Sunflower or Mustard)
2 green chillies slit
2 tablespoons chopped coriander for garnishing

Wash the fish well and fry it lightly to make it firm. Keep aside. Heat the oil in a shallow vessel and fry the curry leaves and onions till golden brown. Add the ginger and garlic paste, chillie powder, cumin powder, coriander powder, turmeric powder and a little water and fry well for some time. Add the Coconut Milk, salt, and a little more water and bring to boil. Add the fish and cook for about 6 to 7 minutes till the fish is firm. Garnish with chopped coriander leaves and slit green chilies Serve with Rice or chapattis.

9. Tangy King Fish / Seer Fish Curry
(In a Tamarind Base)

Serves 6   *Preparation Time 40 minutes*

Ingredients

½ kg sliced King / Seer Fish
3 medium size onions chopped finely
2 tomatoes chopped
2 teaspoons chillie powder
½ teaspoon turmeric powder
1 Cup tamarind juice
1 teaspoon cumin powder
1 teaspoon coriander powder
2 teaspoons chopped garlic
1 teaspoon chopped ginger
4 green chillies slit lengthwise
3 tablespoons Oil
Salt to taste

Wash the fish and marinate it with a pinch of salt and turmeric powder for 15 minutes. Heat oil in suitable vessel and sauté the onions, ginger and garlic for about 5 minutes. Add the tomatoes, chillie powder, cumin powder, coriander powder, turmeric powder, salt and tamarind juice and fry on low heat till the tomatoes are pulpy. Add half cup of water and bring to boil. Add the sliced King Fish / Seer and green chillies and mix gently. Simmer on low heat for about 7 minutes till the fish is cooked. Serve with Rice or bread.

10. Whole Curried Mackerels

Serves 6   Preparation Time 45 minutes

Ingredients

3 medium size mackerels
3 medium size onions chopped finely
2 tomatoes chopped
2 teaspoons chillie powder
½ teaspoon turmeric powder
2 tablespoons Vinegar
2 teaspoons cumin powder
1 teaspoon coriander powder
1 teaspoon ginger and garlic paste
2 green chillies slit lengthwise
3 tablespoons Oil
Salt to taste

Clean and remove the scales, fins and insides of the mackerels. Marinate with a pinch of salt and turmeric powder for 15 minutes. Heat oil in a flat pan and shallow fry the fish on both sides till evenly brown. Remove and keep aside.

Heat a little more oil in the same pan and sauté the onions till light brown. Add the ginger and garlic paste, tomatoes, chillie powder, cumin powder, coriander powder, turmeric powder, salt and vinegar and fry on low heat till the tomatoes are pulpy. Add one cup of water and bring to boil. Add the mackerels and green chillies and mix gently. Simmer on low heat for about 5 minutes till the fish absorbs the flavours. Serve with Rice or bread.

11. Fried Mackerels

Serves 6   Preparation Time 45 minutes

Ingredients

6 medium size mackerels
3 tablespoons oil
3 teaspoons chillie powder
2 teaspoons ginger garlic paste
1 teaspoon cumin powder
½ teaspoon coriander powder
½ teaspoon turmeric powder
2 teaspoons lime juice or vinegar
1 teaspoon salt

Clean and remove the scales, fins and insides of the fish. Wash well. Mix all the above ingredients together with a little water to form a paste. Slit each mackerel lengthwise on either side keeping the center bone intact. Stuff the paste into each mackerel evenly on either side of the center bone. Rub some of the paste on the outsides as well. Keep aside for about 30 minutes. Heat oil in a flat pan and shallow fry the fish on both sides till evenly brown. Serve with White Steamed rice and Pepper Water.

12. Simple Fried Fish

Serves 6   Preparation Time 45 minutes

Ingredients

6 slices of any good fleshy fish
2 teaspoons chillie powder
1 teaspoon turmeric powder
Salt to taste
4 tablespoons oil for frying

Wash the fish and coat it with the chillie powder, salt and turmeric powder. Heat oil in a flat pan and shallow fry the pieces about 3 at a time, till nice and brown on both sides. Serve with bread and chips. This is also a good accompaniment to pepper water and rice.

13. Green Masala Fried Fish

Serves 6   Preparation Time 1 hour

Ingredients

1 kg good fleshy fish cut into thick slices
2 teaspoons ginger garlic paste
3 tablespoons coriander leaves
1 teaspoon cumin powder
3 green chillies
¼ teaspoon turmeric powder
Salt to taste
4 tablespoons oil
2 tablespoons vinegar

Grind the green chillies and green coriander together to a paste. Mix in the cumin powder, ginger garlic paste, salt, turmeric powder and vinegar. Marinate the fish slices with this paste and keep aside for half an hour. Heat oil in a flat pan and shallow fry the Fish on both sides till brown. Serve with Rice and Pepper water or Bread.

14. Red Masala Fried Fish

Serves 6   Preparation Time 1 hour

Ingredients

1 kg good fleshy fish cut into thick slices
2 teaspoons ginger garlic paste
2 tablespoons red chillie powder
1 teaspoon cumin powder
½ teaspoon turmeric powder
1 teaspoon spice powder or garam masala
1 teaspoon coriander powder
Salt to taste
6 tablespoons oil
2 tablespoons vinegar

Mix all the ingredients together (except the oil) with a little water. Marinate the fish with this paste and keep aside for 1 hour. Heat oil in a shallow pan and fry the fish on both sides till brown. Use a little more oil if necessary. Serve with bread or with Rice.

15. Black Pepper Fish Fry

Serves 6   Preparation Time 1 hour

Ingredients

1 kg good fleshy fish cut into thick slices
1 tablespoon Black Pepper Powder
¼ teaspoon Turmeric powder
1teaspoon chillie powder
1 teaspoon coriander powder
Salt to taste
Oil for frying
2 tablespoons lime juice
8 curry leaves

Marinate the fish slices with the pepper powder, chillie powder, turmeric powder, coriander powder, salt, lime juice and curry leaves for about half and hour.Heat oil in a Flat pan or Griddle and shallow fry the marinated fish till brown. The curry leaves will also shrivel up and give the fish a nice flavour. Serve with rice or bread.

16. Lemony Fish Fry

Serves 6   Preparation Time 30 minutes

Ingredients

6 slices of any good fleshy fish
2 tablespoons oil
Salt to taste
1 teaspoon chillie powder
½ teaspoon turmeric powder
2 teaspoon lime / lemon juice

Marinate the fish with the salt, chillie powder and turmeric powder for about 15 minutes. Heat oil in a suitable pan and shallow fry the fish till done. Sprinkle the lime / lemon juice over the cooked fish while still hot. Serve with Steamed rice or Bread.

17. Fried Fish Roe

Serves 6   Preparation Time 30 minutes

Ingredients

½ kg Fish Roe
2 teaspoons pepper powder
3 tablespoons oil or butter
2 onions chopped finely

Salt to taste
2 green chillies chopped finely

Wash and cut the Fish Roe into thick slices about an inch in thickness. Coat it with the salt and pepper. Heat oil or butter in a pan till smoky and fry the onions and green chillies till golden. Add the fish Roe and fry till brown. It will taste like scrambled eggs.

18. Shark Fish Vindaloo

Serves 6   Preparation Time 45 minutes

Ingredients

½ kg shark fish cut into medium size pieces
2 medium sized onions chopped
2 teaspoons chillie powder
2 teaspoons cumin powder
2 teaspoons garlic paste
2 tablespoons vinegar
Salt to taste
2 tomatoes pureed or chopped finely
2 tablespoons oil

Heat oil in a pan and add the onions and fry till light brown. Add the garlic paste and sauté for a while. Add the chillie powder, cumin powder, tomato puree and salt and fry for some time. Add the shark pieces and the vinegar and mix well. Add a just a little more water and cook till the gravy is slightly thick. Serve with rice or bread.

19. Shark Mince Fry (Shark Puttu)

Serves 6   Preparation Time 45 minutes

Ingredients

1 kg shark fish without the skin and bones cut into pieces
3 onions minced well
2 green chilies minced
2-teaspoons chillie powder
½ teaspoon turmeric powder
1 teaspoon cumin powder
2 teaspoons ginger garlic paste
4 tablespoons oil
Salt to taste

Wash the shark pieces well then boil in a little water with a pinch of turmeric and a little salt till soft. Drain the water, and crumble into mince when slightly cold. Heat oil in a pan and fry the onions till golden brown. Add the garlic ginger paste, green chillies, chillie powder, cumin powder and turmeric powder and fry for a few minutes till the oil separates. Now add the boiled shark mince and mix well. Add salt to taste. Cook on low heat turning all the time till it turns a nice brown colour. Serve with bread or rice.

20. Fried Salt Fish

Serves 6   Preparation Time 30 minutes

Ingredients

4 or 5 pieces of good salt fish or Bombay Duck
2 teaspoons chillie powder
½ teaspoon turmeric powder
½ teaspoon cumin powder
4 tablespoons oil

127

Soak the salt fish in a little water for about 15 minutes then wash well. Mix in the chillie powder, turmeric powder, cumin powder and salt. Heat the oil in a flat pan and fry the salt fish pieces till nice and brown.

---

21. Salt Fish / Dry Fish Curry

Serves 6   Preparation Time 45 minutes

Ingredients

6 to 8 pieces of any good Salt Fish or Bombay Duck
½ cup thick tamarind juice extracted from a lime size ball of tamarind
2 big onions chopped finely
1 tablespoon ginger garlic paste
3 teaspoons chillie powder
1 teaspoon cumin powder
2 teaspoons coriander powder
½ teaspoon turmeric powder
Salt to taste
3 tablespoons oil
2 tomatoes chopped
2 green chillies slit lengthwise
2 tablespoons chopped coriander leaves for garnishing

Wash the Salt Fish well and soak for about 1 hour in a little water. Rinse the pieces well to remove any sandy residue. Fry the salt fish or Bombay Duck lightly with a little oil to make it firm. Heat the oil in a shallow vessel and fry the onions till golden brown. Add the ginger garlic paste, chillie powder, cumin powder, coriander powder, turmeric powder, chopped tomatoes and a little water and fry well for some time. Add the salt, tamarind juice and a little more water if gravy is required and bring to boil. Add the salt fish and simmer for about 5 minutes for the salt fish to absorb the gravy. Garnish with chopped coriander leaves and slit green chilies.

22. Dry Shrimp Curry

Serves 6   Preparation Time 45 minutes

Ingredients

300 grams dry Shrimps / Prawns
3 tomatoes chopped
3 onions sliced finely
2 teaspoons chillie powder
½ teaspoon turmeric powder
1 teaspoon cumin powder
1 teaspoon coriander powder (optional)
Salt to taste
1 teaspoon ginger and garlic paste
3 tablespoons oil
2 tablespoons vinegar

Soak the dry shrimps / prawns in water for half an hour, then wash well to remove any sandy residue. Marinate the shrimps / prawns with the chillie powder, turmeric powder, cumin powder, coriander powder, vinegar and salt and keep aside for 15 minutes.

Heat oil in a pan and fry the onions till golden brown. Add the garlic paste, ginger paste and tomatoes and fry till the tomatoes turn pulpy. Add the marinated prawns / shrimps and mix well. Add 1 cup of water and cook on medium heat for about 20 minutes till the prawns / shrimps are cooked. Serve with rice, Bread or Chapattis.

23. Fish Cutlets

Serves 6 *Preparation Time 45 minutes*

Ingredients

3 potatoes boiled. peeled and mashed well
½ Kg of any flesh fish without the bones
2 green chilies chopped finely
1 teaspoon pepper powder
2 teaspoons chopped coriander leaves
1 egg beaten well
3 tablespoons breadcrumbs
3 tablespoons oil
Salt to taste

Boil the fish in a little water and a little salt for about 5 minutes. Remove from heat and cool. Crumble the fish with a fork and mix it together with the potatoes, green chilies, pepper powder, salt and coriander leaves. Form into cutlets. Heat the oil in a flat pan. When hot dip each cutlet into the beaten egg, roll in breadcrumbs and shallow fry on low heat on both sides till brown. Serve with rice and dhal or pepper water. These cutlets could also be served as starters at a party.

24. Fish Croquettes

Serves 6 *Preparation Time 45 minutes*

Ingredients

300 grams good fleshy fish fillets
2 teaspoons chopped mint
1 teaspoon pepper powder
Salt to taste
2 tablespoons tomato sauce
1 teaspoon butter

1 egg beaten
Yolk of one egg
3 tablespoons oil
3 tablespoons bread crumbs
1 cup boiled and mashed potatoes

Wash the fish and cook in a little water with some salt till soft. Remove from the heat and cool. When cold mash the fish with a fork. Mix in the mashed potatoes, mint, pepper, salt, tomato sauce, butter and the egg yolk. Form into croquettes (cigar shape). Heat oil in a flat pan. Dip each croquette in the beaten egg, roll in bread crumbs then shallow fry on all sides till brown. Drain and serve with tartar sauce.

Note: 1 tin of Tuna Fish can be used instead of the fresh fish to make Tuna Fish Croquettes.

25. Fish and Potato Cutlets

Serves 6   *Preparation Time 1 hour*

Ingredients

300 grams good fleshy fish fillets
2 teaspoons chopped mint
1 teaspoon pepper powder
Salt to taste
2 tablespoons tomato sauce
2 green chillies chopped finely
1 teaspoon butter
1 egg beaten
3 tablespoons oil
3 tablespoons bread crumbs
1 cup boiled and mashed potatoes

Wash the fish and cook in a little water with some salt till soft. Remove from the heat and cool. When cold mash the fish with a fork. Mix in the mashed potatoes, mint, pepper, salt, chillies, tomato sauce and butter. Divide into equal portions. Pat into oval shapes and flatten with a knife. Now heat the oil in a flat pan. Dip each cutlet in the beaten egg, then shallow fry on both sides till brown. Serve as a side dish or a snack.

26. Shark Mince Cutlets

Serves 6   Preparation Time 45 minutes

Ingredients

½ kg shark fish (without the skin) cut into medium size pieces
3 Potatoes boiled and mashed
1 teaspoon chillie powder
½ teaspoon spice powder / garam masala powder
2 green chilies minced
2 tablespoons chopped coriander leaves
1 egg beaten well
3 tablespoons breadcrumbs
3 tablespoons oil
Salt to taste

Boil the shark with a little water and a pinch of salt for about 6 minutes. Drain the soup and remove the bones. Mix the boiled shark together with the potatoes, green chilies, chillie powder, spice / garam masala powder, salt and coriander leaves. Form into oval shapes and flatten on top. Heat oil in a pan. When hot dip each cutlet into the beaten egg, roll into the breadcrumbs and shallow fry on low heat on both sides till brown. Serve as a snack or a side dish with rice and pepper water.

27. Steamed Fish and Potato Mash

Serves 6   *Preparation Time 45 minutes*

Ingredients

3 boiled potatoes mash well
1 cup of boiled fish without bones
2 onions minced well
2 green chilies minced
1-teaspoon pepper powder
2 tablespoons chopped coriander leaves
2 eggs beaten well
3 tablespoons breadcrumbs
3 tablespoons oil
Salt to taste
2 teaspoons tomato sauce
2 teaspoons butter

Mix the fish together with the potatoes and all the other ingredients. Place this mixture in flat pan. Brush all over with the remaining beaten egg on top. Steam this mixture in a suitable pan or a pressure cooker for about 15 minutes. Serve hot with bread.

28. Temperado Prawns (Tempered Prawns)

The word 'Temperado' a Portuguese word which literally means to sauté or fry. This is a semi-dry curry and the gravy clings thickly to the prawns, imbuing them with intense, sweet-sharp, hot flavours.

Serves 6   *Preparation Time 45 minutes*

Ingredients

½ kg good prawns cleaned and de-veined
1 teaspoon lime / lemon juice

Salt to taste
2 onions chopped finely
1 teaspoon finely chopped garlic
1 teaspoon finely chopped root ginger
2 tablespoons Oil
¼ teaspoon turmeric powder
1 teaspoon cumin powder
½ teaspoon garam masala powder / all spice powder
2 teaspoon chillie powder
2 tablespoons tomato paste
2 tablespoons chopped coriander leaves

Marinate the prawns with the lime juice, turmeric and salt for 15 minutes. Fry the onion, garlic and ginger gently in the oil until golden brown. Now add the chillie powder, cumin powder, garam masala / all spice powder and fry for a few minutes. Add the prawns and sauté for around 3 minutes until the prawns start to turn pink. Now add the tomato paste and cook on low heat for about 5 more minutes. Garnish with fresh coriander and serve with bread, rice or chapattis.

29. Prawn Moilee

Serves 6   Preparation Time 45 minutes

Ingredients

500 grams cleaned and de-veined prawns
1 teaspoon ginger garlic paste
¼ teaspoon turmeric powder
5 tablespoons coconut milk
2 tablespoons oil
1 teaspoon pepper powder
4 green chillies slit lengthwise
Salt to taste
2 onions sliced finely
2 small tomatoes chopped into quarters

Heat the oil in a pan and sauté the onions till golden brown. Add the ginger garlic paste and fry for a few minutes. Add the prawns, coconut milk, green chillies, pepper powder, turmeric powder, tomatoes and salt and mix well. Add 1 cup of water and cook on medium heat till the prawns are tender. Serve with rice or hoppers.

30. Spicy Prawn Curry

Serves 6   *Preparation Time 1 hour*

Ingredients

500 grams cleaned and de-veined prawns
1 teaspoon cumin seeds
2 green chillies slit lengthwise
1 teaspoon ginger and garlic paste
3 tomatoes chopped
2 onions sliced finely
1 teaspoon spice powder or garam masala powder
2 teaspoon chillie powder
2 tablespoons coconut paste / coconut milk
3 tablespoons oil
Salt to taste

Heat oil in a suitable pan and add the cumin seeds. When they begin to splutter add the onions and fry till golden brown. Add the prawns and stir fry for a few minutes till they change colour. Now add all the other ingredients and a little water and stir well. Simmer on low heat till the prawns are cooked and the gravy is thick. Serve with rice, chapattis or bread.

31. Prawn Vindaloo

Serves 6   Preparation Time 45 minutes

Ingredients

½ kg fresh prawns shelled and de-veined
2 medium sized onions chopped
2 teaspoons chillie powder
2 teaspoons cumin powder
2 teaspoons garlic paste
2 tablespoons vinegar
Salt to taste
2 tomatoes pureed or chopped finely
2 tablespoons oil

Wash the prawns well and keep aside. Heat oil in a pan and add the onions and fry till light brown. Add the garlic paste and sauté for a while. Add the chillie powder, cumin powder, tomato and salt and fry for some time. Add the prawns and the vinegar and mix well. Add a little more water and cook till the gravy is slightly thick and the prawns are cooked. Serve with rice or bread.

32. Green Masala Prawns

Serves 6   Preparation Time 45 minutes

Ingredients

½ kg medium size prawns cleaned and de-veined
2 teaspoons ginger garlic paste
4 green chilies
3 tablespoons coriander leaves
1 teaspoon cumin seeds
2 cloves, 2 cardamom,2 pieces of cinnamon
½ teaspoon turmeric powder

Salt to taste
3 tablespoons oil
2 onions sliced finely
½ cup coconut paste

Grind the green chilies, coriander leaves, coconut, cinnamon, cloves, cardamom and cumin seeds to a smooth paste in a blender. Heat oil in a pan and fry the onions till golden brown. Add the ginger garlic paste and turmeric powder and fry for some time. Now add the ground masala and salt and mix well. Keep frying on low heat till the oil separates from the mixture. Add the prawns and sufficient water to cover the prawns and cook for 5 to 6 minutes. Serve hot.

---

33. Prawns and Brinjal Curry

Serves 6   *Preparation Time 1 hour*

Ingredients

½ kg prawns cleaned and de-veined
4 medium size round Brinjals / Eggplants
½ teaspoon turmeric powder
2 teaspoons chillie powder
1 teaspoon cumin powder
1 teaspoon coriander powder
3 tomatoes chopped
3 onions chopped finely
Salt to taste
3 tablespoons oil
2 teaspoons ginger garlic paste

Wash the prawns well. Cut the brinjals into quarters and soak in water. Heat one tablespoon oil in a pan and add the prawns and a pinch of turmeric and stir fry till the prawns are half cooked and the water dries up. Keep aside. In the same pan add the remaining oil and fry the onions till golden brown. Now add the chopped tomatoes and ginger garlic paste and sauté till the tomatoes are reduced to pulp. Add the chillie powder, turmeric powder, salt, coriander powder and cumin powder and mix well. Drop in the brinjals and the cooked prawns and stir-fry for a few minutes. Add a little water and simmer for 10 minutes till the gravy is thick.

Note: *The same Prawn Curry could be cooked with Fenugreek / Methi leaves, Ridge Gourd, Zucchini, Gherkins, etc*

---

34. Spicy Prawns Fry

Serves 6   Preparation Time 45 minutes

Ingredients

½ kg medium sized prawns cleaned and de-veined
2 teaspoons chillie powder
1 teaspoon turmeric powder
1 teaspoon cumin powder
2 onions sliced finely
Salt to taste
4 tablespoons oil
2 tablespoons chopped coriander leaves for garnishing

Wash the prawns well and mix in the chillie powder, turmeric powder, cumin powder and salt. Heat the oil in a large pan and sauté the onions for some time.Add the marinated prawns and mix well. Add a little water and cook on low heat till the prawns are cooked. Keep frying till all the water dries up. Garnish with chopped coriander leaves.

35. Prawn Pepper Fry

Serves 6   *Preparation Time 45 minutes*

Ingredients

1 kg medium sized prawns cleaned and de-veined
2 teaspoons fresh ground pepper powder
½ teaspoon turmeric powder
1 teaspoon coriander powder
1 tablespoon chopped garlic
2 onions chopped
Salt to taste
4 tablespoons oil

Wash and de-vein the prawns and marinate it with the pepper powder, turmeric powder, coriander powder and salt. Heat the oil in a large pan and sauté the onions and chopped garlic for a few minutes. Add the marinated prawns and mix well. Add a little water and cook on low heat till the prawns are cooked. Keep frying till all the water dries up. Serve with bread or rice.

36. Batter Fried Prawns

Serves 6   *Preparation time 45 minutes*

Ingredients

½ kg medium size prawns
4 tablespoons plain flour or maida
2 teaspoons chillie powder
½ teaspoon turmeric powder
Salt to taste
1 egg beaten
Oil as required for deep frying

Wash, clean and de-vein the pawns. Make a batter with the flour, chillie powder, salt, turmeric beaten egg and a little water. The batter should not be too thick or too thin. Dip the prawns in the batter and deep fry till golden brown. Serve as a side dish or a snack.

---

37. Simple Crab Curry

Serves 6   *Preparation Time 45 minutes*

Ingredients

6 to 8 medium sized crabs or 5 big ones cleaned and shelled
2 big onions sliced finely
2 teaspoons coriander powder
2 teaspoons chillie powder
2 teaspoons ginger and garlic paste
Salt to taste
2 or 3 tablespoons oil
½ teaspoon turmeric powder
½ teaspoon all spice powder or garam masala powder

Clean and wash the crabs well and keep aside. Heat oil in a pan and sauté the onions and ginger garlic paste for some time. Add the chillie powder, coriander powder, turmeric powder, all spice powder / garam masala power, salt and a little water and fry till the mixture separates from the oil. Now add the crabs and mix well. Add a little water. Cover and cook on low heat for about 10 minutes till the gravy is very thick. Serve with bread or rice.

38. Crabs In Coconut Milk Curry

Serves 6   *Preparation Time 45 minutes*

Ingredients

6 to 8 medium sized crabs or 5 big ones cleaned and shelled
2 big onions sliced finely
1 teaspoon coriander powder
2 teaspoons chillie powder
2 teaspoons ginger garlic paste
Salt to taste
3 tablespoons oil
½ teaspoon turmeric powder
1 teaspoon cumin powder
1 cup coconut paste or coconut milk
2 tomatoes chopped finely

Wash the crabs well and keep aside. Heat oil in a pan and sauté the onions and ginger garlic paste for some time. Add the chopped tomatoes chillie powder, cumin powder, coriander powder, turmeric powder, salt and a little water and fry till the mixture separates from the oil. Now add the crabs, coconut milk and mix well. Cover and cook on low heat for about 10 minutes till dry. Serve with bread or rice

39. Crab Vindaloo

Serves 6   *Preparation Time 45 minutes*

Ingredients

6 to 8 medium sized crabs or 5 big ones cleaned and shelled
2 medium sized onions chopped
2 teaspoons chillie powder
2 teaspoons cumin powder
2 teaspoons garlic paste

2 tablespoons vinegar
Salt to taste
2 tomatoes pureed or chopped finely
2 tablespoons oil

Heat oil in a pan and add the onions and fry till light brown. Add the garlic paste and sauté for a while. Add the chillie powder, cumin powder, tomato puree and salt and fry for some time. Add the crabs and the vinegar and mix well. Add a just a little more water and cook till the gravy is slightly thick.

---

40. Spicy Pepper Crabs

Serves 6   Preparation Time 45 minutes

Ingredients

6 to 8 medium sized crabs or 5 big ones cleaned and shelled
2 teaspoons ground pepper powder
1 teaspoon turmeric powder
1 teaspoon coriander powder
2 onions sliced finely
2 green chillies slit lengthwise
Salt to taste
4 tablespoons oil

Marinate the crabs with the pepper powder, turmeric powder, coriander powder and salt. Keep aside for 15 minutes. Meanwhile, heat the oil in a large pan and sauté the onions for some time Add the green chillies and fry for 2 minutes. Add the marinated crabs and mix well. Add a little water and cook on low heat till the prawns are cooked. Keep frying till all the water dries up.

2.
PEPPER WATER, SOUPS
AND MULLIGATAWNY

---

1. Anglo-Indian Pepper Water

Pepper water or Rasam invariably forms part of the afternoon meal. It is usually had with plain white rice and accompanied by meat, poultry, or a seafood dish that is generally a dry fry. Pepper water should always be of a watery consistency. Many people like to drink a cup of pepper water after a meal since it aids in digestion.

Serves 6   Preparation Time 20 minutes

Ingredients

2 large tomatoes chopped
1 teaspoon pepper powder
1 teaspoon chillie powder
1 teaspoon cumin powder
½ teaspoon turmeric powder
½ teaspoon coriander powder
Salt to taste
½ cup tamarind juice extracted from a small ball of tamarind or 2 teaspoons tamarind paste

Cook all the above with 3 or 4 cups of water in a vessel on high heat till it boils. Reduce the heat and cook on low heat for about 5 or 6 minutes. Season as follows with the under mentioned ingredients which should be used whenever a dish is to be seasoned/ tempered.

143

FOR THE SEASONING:

I small onion sliced
2 red chilies broken into bits
1 teaspoon chopped garlic crushed roughly
½ teaspoon mustard seeds
A few curry leaves
2 teaspoons oil

Heat the oil in a sutiable vessel and add the mustard seeds. When they begin to splutter, add the curry leaves, onion, crushed garlic and red chilies and sauté for a few minutes. Pour the cooked pepper water into this and simmer for 2 minutes. Turn off the heat. Serve hot with rice and any meat side dish.

Note: The pepper water can be prepared by using fresh red chilies, cumin seeds, coriander seeds and peppercorns ground in a mixer or blender instead of the powders.

2. DHAL PEPPER WATER
(LENTILS BASED PEPPER WATER)

Serves 6   Preparation Time 45 minutes

Ingredients

1 Cup Tur Dhal
2 cups of water
1onion chopped
2 teaspoons chillie powder
1large tomato chopped
1 teaspoon cumin powder
1 teaspoon pepper powder
1 tablespoon garlic paste
½ teaspoon turmeric powder
1 teaspoon coriander powder

½ cup tamarind juice extracted from a small ball of tamarind or 2 teaspoons tamarind paste
Salt to taste

Cook the Tur dhal with 2 cups of water till the dhal is cooked. Add the chillie powder, tomato, cumin powder, pepper powder, garlic paste, turmeric powder, coriander powder, tamarind juice, salt and some more water to the cooked dhal and bring to boil. Cook on low heat for a few more minutes. Season with mustered seeds, curry leaves and crushed garlic.

---

3. Breast Bone Pepper Water

Serves 6   preparation Time 45 minutes

Ingredients

½ kg soup bones and pieces of meat preferably from the breast portion
2 teaspoons cumin powder
2 teaspoons chillie powder
1 teaspoon pepper powder
2 teaspoons coriander powder
½ teaspoon turmeric powder
2 large onions chopped
2 large tomatoes chopped
Salt to taste
1 teaspoon crushed garlic
½ cup tamarind juice
½ cup coconut paste or coconut milk (optional)
2 tablespoons chopped coriander leaves for garnishing

Cook all the above ingredients with about 6 cups of water in a pressure cooker first on high heat then on low for ½ an hour till the meat and bones are soft and the pepper water is quite thick. Season with mustard, curry leaves and chopped onion.

Garnish with coriander leaves. Serve hot with plain rice and any chutney.

---

4. Horse Gram Pepper Water

Serves 6   Preparation Time 50 minutes

Ingredients

1 cup of horse gram
2 teaspoons chillie powder
2 teaspoons cumin powder
2 teaspoons pepper powder
1 teaspoon garlic paste
1 teaspoon coriander powder
1 cup tamarind juice
½ teaspoon turmeric powder
Salt to taste

For the seasoning:

3 pods garlic crushed, 2 red chilies broken into bits,1/2 teaspoon mustard seeds, a few curry leaves, 1 small onion sliced, and 1 tablespoon oil.

Soak the horse gram in water for a few hours. Wash well then pressure cook it with 2 cups of water and ½ teaspoon turmeric powder till soft. Add the chillie powder, cumin powder, coriander powder, pepper powder, garlic paste, tamarind juice and salt and some more water and cook for 10 minutes on low heat. In another vessel heat the oil, then add the curry leaves, crushed garlic, red chillie, mustard seeds and the sliced onion and sauté till the onions and garlic turn brown and the mustard seeds splutter. Pour the Horse Gram Pepper Water mixture into this seasoning. Add more water if required. Serve hot with plain rice and coconut chutney.

5. Dry Shrimp Pepper Water

Serves 6   Preparation Time 30 minutes

Ingredients

1 teaspoon chillie powder
1 teaspoon cumin powder
1 teaspoon pepper powder
½ teaspoon turmeric powder
2 tomatoes chopped
½ cup tamarind juice
Salt to taste
2 teaspoons dried shrimp powder

Puree the tomatoes and add 3 cups of water. Now add all the other ingredients except the shrimp powder. Boil for 10 minutes. Season the pepper water with mustard seeds, curry leaves, 2 red chilies broken into bits and half an onion chopped. Add the shrimp powder and mix well. Serve Hot with rice.

6. Meat And Vegetable Broth

Serves 6   Preparation time 1 hour

Ingredients

½ kg marrow bones (beef or mutton)
4 to 6 cups of water
Salt and Pepper to taste
2 carrots
6 to 8 string beans
1 medium size onion
1 large tomato chopped

Wash and cut the carrots, beans, onion, tomato and any other vegetables of your choice into suitable sizes. Place the bones and vegetables in a large vessel or pot. Add sufficient water, salt and pepper and simmer on low heat for at least one hour or till the soup is quite thick and and gives out a nice aroma. Serve hot.

---

7. Beef And Cabbage Soup

Serves 6   Preparation 2 hours

Ingredients

½ kg beef with bones cut into medium size pieces
1 medium size cabbage coarsely cut
3 tomatoes chopped
2 onions chopped thickly
2 teaspoons pepper powder
Salt to taste
1 teaspoon chopped garlic
2 teaspoons chopped mint
2 litres of water

Boil all the above ingredients together in a suitable pot or pan on high heat for some time. Lower heat and simmer till the meat is well cooked and the broth is thick and a good brown colour. Serve with Bread or Buns.

---

8. Ox Tail Soup

Serves 6   Preparation Time 2 hours

Ingredients

1 oxtail chopped into medium size pieces
4 carrots peeled and chopped
3 onions chopped
2 litres water
2 teaspoons pepper powder

Salt to taste
2 teaspoons butter
2 teaspoons chopped mint leaves
2 tomatoes chopped
1 green chillie

Heat the butter in a suitable pan or crock pot. Fry the onions and carrots till light brown. Add the tomatoes and sauté for a few minutes till pulpy. Now add all the other ingredients and sufficient water. Cook on high heat for some time, then simmer on low heat till the soup is thick and the oxtail is tender and soft. Serve with fried bread.

9. Beef Shin Bone Soup

Serves 6   Preparation Time 2 hours

Ingredients

½ kg Beef Shin Bones chopped into medium size pieces
2 teaspoons pepper powder
2 teaspoons chopped mint
2 large tomatoes chopped
2 onions sliced thickly
Salt to taste

Wash the Shin Bones thoroughly, and boil with all the other ingredients in sufficient water for about one hour till the soup is thick. Add more salt and pepper if needed. Serve with bread.

10. Trotters Soup

Serves 6   Preparation time 30 minutes

Ingredients

6 to 8 trotters (mutton or pork) each to be chopped into 2 pieces
2 or 3 green chilies (optional)
Salt to taste
2 teaspoons pepper powder
1 tomato chopped
1 large onion chopped

Wash the trotters well. Place all the above ingredients together with the trotters and about 3 or 4 glasses of water in a pressure cooker. Pressure cook for about 20 minutes or till the trotters are tender and the soup is thick. Serve hot. This is a very nourishing soup.

11. Simple Chicken Soup

Serves 6   Preparation Time 2 hours

Ingredients

½ kg chicken cut into medium size pieces
2 onions chopped thickly
2 tomatoes chopped
2 teaspoons pepper powder
Salt to taste
1 bay leaf
1 teaspoon chopped garlic
1 teaspoon chopped mint leaves

Place all the above ingredients in a suitable vessel or pot with 8 to 10 cups of water and bring to boil. Reduce heat and simmer for about 1 hour till the chicken is soft and tender and the soup thickens. Serve with steamed rice or bread. This soup is excellent when you have a cold.

12. Lamb Mulligatawny Soup

Serves 6   Preparation time 30 minutes

Ingredients

1 kg lamb or mutton with bones preferably from the breast portion
1 handful Masoor dhal (Red Gram Dhal)
2 cups coconut milk
2 tablespoons oil
3 green chilies
2 teaspoons red chillie powder
1 teaspoon coriander powder
½ teaspoon turmeric powder
1 teaspoon cumin powder
1 tablespoon ginger garlic paste
1 tablespoon lime juice
Salt to taste
8 to 10 curry leaves
2 medium size onions sliced
2 tablespoons chopped mint for garnishing

Cook the meat and dhal with sufficient water till tender. Whisk till the dhal is smooth. Heat oil in a big pan and fry the curry leaves, green chilies and onions till slightly brown. Add the ginger garlic paste and sauté for a few minutes. Now add the chillie powder, cumin powder, coriander powder and turmeric and fry for a few minutes till the oil separates from the mixture. Mix in the cooked mutton and dhal and mix well. Slowly add the coconut milk and salt to taste. Add 2 more cups of water and simmer for about 15 to 20 minutes. Remove from heat and add the lime juice. Garnish with mint leaves. Serve as a soup or with bread or rice.

---

13. Chicken Mulligatawny Soup

Serves 6   Preparation time 45 minutes

Ingredients

½ kg chicken chopped into medium size pieces
1 teaspoon chillie powder
2 teaspoons pepper powder
1 teaspoon cumin powder
1 teaspoon coriander powder
1teaspoon crushed garlic
2 big onions sliced
1 cup coconut paste or coconut milk
1 tablespoon vinegar
2 Bay leaves
2 pieces cinnamon bark (about one inch in size)
Salt to taste
1 tablespoon chopped fresh mint for garnishing

Cook the chicken and all the ingredients with 6 to 8 cups of water in a large vessel on high heat till it reaches boiling point. Lower the heat and simmer for at least one hour till the soup is nice and thick. Garnish with mint leaves. Serve with bread or rice.

---

14. Dal Mulligatawny Soup

Serves 6   Preparation Time 1 hour

Ingredients:

1 cup masoor dhal
3 onions sliced

3 tomatoes chopped
1 teaspoon chillie powder
1 teaspoon ginger and garlic paste
1 teaspoon pepper powder / ground pepper
Salt to taste
1 Bay leaf
1small stick cinnamon
3 cloves

Cook the masoor dhal with 4 cups of water together with the tomato ginger and garlic paste, onion, pepper powder, bay leaf, chillie powder, cinnamon, cloves and salt till soft. Remove and cool well. Grind in a blender and strain through a sieve. Add a little more water if the soup is too thick. Heat again and add the butter and serve hot with rolls or crotons.

---

15. Anglo-Burmese Khow Suey

Anglo-Burmese Khow Suey is not exactly a Soup but is close enough to classify as a one dish meal.

This Anglicized Burmese dish is a wonderful, delicious, mouth watering concoction of noodles, spicy chicken curry and lots of toppings. While the noodles and chicken curry form the base of this dish, it allows each one to choose their own toppings. As the name suggests, it is a Burmese dish, but was brought into Eastern India when many Indians fled from Burma and crossed over into India during World War II. It is a very popular dish with Anglo-Indians living in Calcuta and Eastern India.

Serves 6   Preparation time 45 minutes

Ingredients:

1 kg Chicken boiled and shredded (discard bones)
1 teaspoon whole black pepper corns
2 Bay leaves
2 pieces cinnamon bark (about one inch in size)

Salt to taste
2 medium sized onions chopped fine
2 teaspoons garlic and ginger paste
1 teaspoon chillie powder
1 cup cooked and mashed Moong Dhal (yellow split lentils)
2 tablespoons fish sauce (optional)
2 teaspoons coriander powder
1 teaspoon cumin powder
1 teaspoon garam masala / all spice powder
2 teaspoons chillie powder
1 cup coconut milk
500 grams thin egg noodles

For the garnish:

1 cup spring onions chopped fine
2 onions sliced finely and fried golden brown
4 tablespoons chopped garlic fried in oil
1 cup boiled eggs chopped into tiny pieces
5 tablespoons dry prawn powder (make by coarsely grinding dry prawns)
1 cup chopped coriander leaves
Juice of 1 lemon

Heat 2 tablespoons oil in a deep heavy-bottomed pan and sauté the onions, black pepper corns, bay leaves, and cinnamon sticks till the onions turn golden brown. Add the ginger and garlic paste and fry for 2 minutes. Add the shredded chicken, coriander powder, cumin powder, red chillie powder and garam masala / spice powder and fry for another 5 minutes. Mix in the cooked moong dhal / lentil paste, coconut milk, fish sauce and salt and cook for about 5 minutes. Keep aside.

Boil the noodles in sufficient water with a little salt. Strain and run cold water over them. Pour 1 tablespoon of oil over the noodles to keep them from sticking, and toss to mix well. Keep aside.

Now heat 3 tablespoons of oil in a small pan till very hot. Turn off the flame and add 1 tbsp of red chillie powder to this oil. Keep this chillie oil aside to cool.

Serve each person individually in deep bowls as follows:

Place a single serving of noodles in each bowl. Top generously with the chicken curry prepared as above. Now top up with the chopped fried garlic, fried onions, chopped spring onion, and boiled egg, one on top of the other as per preference. Drizzle with chillie oil and sprinkle dry prawn powder according to taste. Garnish with chopped coriander leaves. Add a dash of lemon to complete. Have a bowl of chopped green chillies in vinegar as an accompaniment

Note: *The Khowsuey can also be served with plain egg noodles and the chicken curry in a big bowl. The toppings of Fried Garlic, Fried Onions, Chopped Spring onions, Chopped boiled eggs, Chopped green chillies in vinegar,Lime wedges and Ground dry shrimp powder could be served in small bowls and each person could top up their own bowls as per their preference.*

3.
RICE DISHES—
A Rendezvous' With Rice

---

1. Steamed White Rice

Serves 6   *Preparation time 45 minutes*

Ingredients

2 cups rice
4 cups water
A pinch of salt

Wash the rice and soak in 4 cups of water and a pinch of salt for 15 minutes. Place on heat and bring to boil. Reduce heat and cook on low heat till done and all the water is absorbed. Cover and allow to stand for 15 minutes before serving. Serve with any curry, Dhal or pepper water.

This is the standard plain rice eaten every day.

---

2. Yellow Coconut Rice

Serves 6   *Preparation Time 45 minutes*

Ingredients

1 pack of coconut milk diluted with water to get 4 cups of milk or 1 fresh coconut grated and milk extracted to get 4 cups of diluted milk
2 cups of Raw Rice or Basmati Rice
½ teaspoon turmeric powder or a few strands of saffron

Salt to taste
4 tablespoons butter or ghee
3 cloves, 3 cardamoms, 3 small sticks of cinnamon

Heat ghee in a large vessel or Rice cooker and fry the spices for a few minutes. Add the washed rice, salt, turmeric and 4 cups of coconut milk and cook till the rice is done.

Coconut Rice is best eaten with Ball Curry or Chicken curry and Devil Chutney.

3. Lamb / Mutton Biryani

Serves 6   Preparation time 1 hour

Ingredients

1 kg Basmati Rice or any other Good Rice . . . wash and soak
for about 1 hour
1 kg Mutton / Lamb (or Beef) cut into fairly big pieces
3 bay leaves
2 teaspoons all spice powder or garam masala
3 large tomatoes chopped
3 small sticks of cinnamon, 3 cloves, 3 cardamoms
2 cups oil or ghee
Salt to taste
6 green chilies slit lengthwise
3 tablespoons ginger garlic paste
2 teaspoons chillie powder
3 large onions sliced finely
1 teaspoon turmeric powder
½ cup fresh mint leaves
3 tablespoons curds / yogurt

Wash the meat and marinate with the spice powder, green chillies, curds, half the quantity of ginger garlic paste and turmeric powder for half an hour.

Heat the oil or ghee in a large vessel and add the bay leaves, cloves, cinnamon, cardamom, remaining ginger garlic paste and onions and sauté for some time. Add the chopped tomatoes, mint leaves and chillie powder and simmer till the oil separates from the mixture and the tomatoes are reduced to pulp. Add the marinated meat and salt and cook till tender. Remove the pieces and keep aside. Now add sufficient water to the gravy in the vessel so as to get about 7 glasses of liquid. Add the rice and cook till half done. Now add the cooked meat and mix well. Cover and cook on low heat for a few more minutes till all the liquid evaporates and the Biryani is done.

---

4. Jhaldhi Pilaf (Palau) Pilaf in A Hurry

Serves 6   Preparation time 1 hour

Ingredients

2 cups Basmati rice or any other long grained rice
1 cup oil or ghee
2 teaspoons chillie powder
3 big onions sliced finely
3 or 4 green chilies sliced lengthwise
2 tablespoons ginger garlic paste
3 big tomatoes chopped
1 cup ground coconut or 1 pack coconut milk
½ cup fresh mint leaves
½ cup coriander leaves
1 cup curds (yogurt)
½ teaspoon turmeric powder
2 bay leaves
4 cloves, 3 small sticks of cinnamon, 4 cardamoms
Salt to taste

Wash the rice and soak it in a little water for about 20 minutes.

Heat the ghee in a suitable vessel or rice cooker and add the spices and bay leaves and fry for a few minutes. Now add the onions and ginger garlic paste and sauté for some time. Add the turmeric, mint leaves, coriander leaves and chillie powder and fry for a while. Next add the chopped tomatoes and keep on frying till the oil separates from the mixture. Add the curds, slit green chilies, coconut and salt and simmer for a few minutes. Add the rice and 3 cups of water and cook on low heat till done mixing once or twice. Serve with curd chutney and chicken or meat curry.

5. Chicken Biryani

Serves 8W Preparation time 1 hour

Ingredients

1 kg Basmati Rice or any other Good Rice. (wash and soak for about 1 hour)
2 kgs chicken cut into fairly big pieces
3 bay leaves
2 teaspoons spice powder or garam masala
½ kg tomatoes chopped
3 small sticks of cinnamon, 4 cloves, 5 cardamoms
1 nutmeg flower / Star Anise
2 cups oil or ghee
Salt to taste
6 green chilies ground
3 tablespoons ginger garlic paste
2 teaspoons chillie powder
½ kg onions sliced finely
1 teaspoon turmeric powder
½ cup fresh mint leaves
1 cup curds / yogurt

Wash the chicken and marinate with the spice powder, green chillie paste, curds / yogurt, half the quantity of ginger garlic paste and turmeric powder for half an hour.

Heat the oil or ghee in a large vessel and add the cloves, cinnamon, cardamom, nutmeg flower / star Anise, remaining ginger garlic paste and onions and sauté for some time. Add the chopped tomatoes, mint leaves and chillie powder and simmer till the oil separates from the mixture and the tomatoes are reduced to pulp. Add the marinated chicken and salt and cook for 10 minutes till the chicken is done. Remove the chicken pieces and keep aside. Now add sufficient water to the gravy in the vessel so as to get about 7 glasses of liquid. Add the rice and cook till half done. Now add the cooked chicken and mix well. Cover and cook on low heat till all the liquid is absorbed and the Biryani is almost dry. Serve hot with Curd Chutney.

6. Coconut Pilaf (Palau)

Serves 6   Preparation time 45 minutes

Ingredients

1 Fresh coconut scraped and milk extracted to get 4 cups of milk or 1 pack of ready coconut milk diluted to get 4 cups of milk
2 cups of Basmati Rice or any other raw rice
3 green chilies slit lengthwise
2 teaspoons ginger garlic paste
1 teaspoon turmeric powder
Salt to taste
4 tablespoons oil, or ghee or butter
2 onions sliced finely
3 Cardamoms, 2 cloves, 1 stick cinnamon and 1 Bay leaf
1 teaspoon all spice powder / garam masala powder

Heat the oil or ghee in a vessel or rice cooker. Add the Cardamoms, cloves, cinnamon, Bay leaf, onions, ginger garlic paste, green chilies and spice powder and sauté for a few minutes. Now add the turmeric powder, salt, washed rice and 4 cups of coconut milk and cook on low heat till the rice is done. Serve with Ball Curry or Chicken Curry.

---

7. Tomato Pilaf (Palau)

Serves 6   Preparation time 45 minutes

Ingredients

4 large tomatoes pureed and diluted with water to get 3 cups of juice or 1 pack of tomato puree diluted to get 3 cups of juice
3 tablespoons chopped coriander leaves
2 large onions sliced finely
2 cups Raw Rice or Basmati Rice
Salt to taste
2 teaspoons chillie powder
2 teaspoons ginger garlic paste
2 cloves, 3 cardamoms, 2 small sticks of cinnamon
4 tablespoons oil or ghee
2 teaspoons chopped fresh mint

Heat oil in a pan or a rice cooker and sauté the spices, onions, ginger garlic paste and chillie powder for a few minutes. Add the rice, salt, mint, coriander leaves and tomato juice and cook till the rice is done. Serve with salad and Chicken Curry or Pork Vindaloo.

---

8. Plain Pilaf (Palau)

Serves 6   Preparation time 45 minutes

Ingredients

2 cups Basmati Rice or any other rice
2 Bay leaves

4 Cardamoms, 3 Cloves, 1 small stick cinnamon
2 teaspoons ginger garlic paste
Salt to taste
½ cup ghee

Heat the ghee in a pan or rice cooker and fry the bay leaves, and spices for some time. Add the ginger garlic paste and sauté for a few minutes. Add the washed rice and stir fry for 3 or 4 minutes. Add the salt and 4 cups of water and cook till the rice is done. Serve with mutton or pork curry and salad.

---

9. Green Masala Meat Pilaf (Palau)

Serves 6   Preparation time 1 hour

Ingredients

1 kg meat either beef or mutton cut into pieces
½ kg Basmati Rice or any other long grain rice
3 onions sliced finely
2 tablespoons ginger garlic paste
1 cup oil or ghee
3 small sticks of cinnamon, 3 cloves, 3 cardamoms, 2 bay leaves
1 cup coriander leaves chopped
2 tablespoons fresh mint
Salt to taste
3 tablespoons coconut paste
6 green chillies

Wash the meat and boil it with extra water and a little salt till nicely cooked. Remove the meat and keep aside. Grind the coriander leaves, coconut paste and chilies together to a paste.

Heat the oil or ghee in a big vessel and sauté the whole spices, mint, ginger garlic paste and onions till brown. Add the ground paste and fry well. Add sufficient water to the soup to make it 4 cups. Add this to the masala and bring to boil. When boiling, reduce heat and add the rice, salt and cooked meat. Mix well and cook on low heat till done

Note: Chicken can be used instead of meat

---

10. Vegetable Pilaf (Palau)

Serves 6   Preparation time 45 minutes

Ingredients

2 cups basmati rice or any other raw rice — Wash and soak for ½ an hour
3 onions sliced finely
2 cups assorted vegetables such as carrots, beans, peas, cauliflower etc cut into medium size bits
1 cup ground coconut
½ teaspoon turmeric powder
2 teaspoons ginger garlic paste
½ cup oil or ghee
Salt to taste
3 green chilies chopped
2 teaspoons chillie powder
1 teaspoon all spice powder/ garam masala powder
3 tablespoons chopped coriander leaves for garnishing

Heat oil in a suitable vessel or cooker and fry the onions till brown. Add the ginger garlic paste and green chilies and sauté for a few minutes. Add the chopped vegetables, and all the other ingredients and stir-fry for a few minutes till the oil separates from the mixture. Add 3 cups of water and bring to boil. Add the rice and mix well. Cook on medium heat till the rice is cooked and each grain is separate. Garnish with chopped coriander leaves.

11. Prawn Pilaf (Palau)

Serves 6   Preparation time 1 hour

Ingredients

2 cups raw rice — wash and soak for 20 minutes
½ kg cleaned and de-veined prawns
1 cup coconut milk
2 tablespoons ginger garlic paste
2 onions sliced finely
3 green chilies slit lengthwise
2 tablespoons chopped mint leaves
3 tablespoons chopped coriander leaves
1 teaspoon chillie powder
1 teaspoon all spice powder / garam masala powder
½ cup oil or ghee
1 teaspoon coriander powder
Salt to taste

Wash the prawns and keep aside. Heat oil in a vessel and fry the onions till golden brown. Add the ginger garlic paste, green chilies, mint and coriander leaves and sauté for some time. Add the chillie powder, garam masala powder, coriander powder, salt and prawns and mix well. Cook for about 5 minutes on low heat. Add the coconut milk and mix well. Add 3 cups of water and bring to boil. Add the rice and mix well. Cook on low heat till the rice is cooked and all the water dries up. Serve hot with Prawn Vindaloo and salad.

12. Fish Pilaf (Palau)

Serves 6   *Preparation time 1 hour*

Ingredients:

2 cups raw rice (wash and soak for 20 minutes)
1 kg good fleshy fish cut into thick chunks
4 tablespoons coconut paste or 1 cup coconut milk
2 tablespoons ginger garlic paste
3 onions sliced finely
4 green chilies slit lengthwise
2 tablespoon chopped mint leaves
3 tablespoons chopped coriander leaves
3 teaspoons chillie powder
1 teaspoon all spice powder / garam masala powder
½ cup oil
2 tablespoons ghee
1 teaspoon cumin powder
Salt to taste
2 Bay leaves
4 cloves, 2 small sticks of cinnamon, 3 cardamoms
1 teaspoon turmeric powder

Wash the fish and marinate it with a 1 teaspoon chillie powder, ½ teaspoon turmeric powder and a pinch of salt for half and hour. Heat 1 tablespoon oil in a flat pan and lightly fry the fish till firm. Remove and keep aside.

Heat the remaining oil in a suitable vessel and fry the onions, bay leaves and spices till golden brown. Add the ginger garlic paste, green chilies and coriander leaves and sauté for some time. Add all the remaining ingredients. Cook for about 5 minutes on low heat. Add the coconut and mix well. Add 4 cups of water and bring to boil. Add the rice and mix well. Cook on low heat till most of the water has been absorbed. Now mix in the fried fish gently. Simmer till the rice is cooked and all the water dries up. Serve hot with curd and onion chutney.

13. Egg Pilaf (Palau)

Serves 6   *Preparation time 1 hour*

Ingredients

10 Eggs boiled and shelled
½ kg raw rice or Basmati rice
4 tablespoons oil
3 tablespoons ghee
2 teaspoons chillie powder
3 big onions sliced finely
3 or 4 green chilies sliced lengthwise
2 tablespoons ginger garlic paste
2 big tomatoes chopped
4 tablespoons coconut paste or 1 pack coconut milk
½ cup chopped fresh mint leaves
½ cup chopped coriander leaves
1 cup curds (yogurt)
1 teaspoon turmeric powder
2 bay leaves
4 cloves, 3 small sticks of cinnamon, 4 cardamoms
Salt to taste

Wash the rice and soak it in a little water for about 20 minutes. Heat the oil and ghee in a suitable vessel or rice cooker and add the spices and bay leaves and fry for a few minutes. Now add the onions, ginger garlic paste and sauté for some time. Add the turmeric, mint leaves, coriander leaves and chillie powder and fry for a while. Next add the chopped tomatoes and salt and keep on frying till the oil separates from the mixture. Add the boiled eggs, curds, slit green chilies, coconut and salt and simmer for 5 minutes. Add 4 cups of water and bring to boil. Now add the rice and cook on low heat till done, mixing once or twice. Serve with curd chutney and chicken or meat curry.

14. Green Peas Pilaf (Palau)

Serves 6   Preparation time 1 hour

Ingredients

2 cups rice — wash and keep aside
½ cup fresh green peas
3 tablespoons ghee or oil
2 onions sliced finely
2 tomatoes chopped
3 green chillies sliced finely
2 cloves, 3 cardamoms, 2 small sticks of cinnamon
½ teaspoon corriander powder
1 teaspoon all spice powder or garam masala powder
1 teaspoon chillie powder
½ cup chopped coriander leaves
Salt to taste
2 Bay leaves

Heat oil or ghee in a vessel and fry the spices, bay leaves and onions till golden brown. Add the chopped tomatoes, green chillies, spice powder, coriander powder chillie powder and peas and cook till the tomatoes turn to pulp. Add the rice, salt and chopped coriander leaves and mix well. Add 4 cups of water and cook on medium heat till the rice is done and all the water dries up. Serve with salad and any curry.

Note: Mutton or chicken can be added if desired

---

15. Anglo-Indian Pish-Pash
(A Simple Rice And Lentils Mix Up)

Serves 6   *Preparation time 1 hour*

Ingredients

1 cup raw rice – wash and keep aside
¼ cup Masur Dhal or Moong Dhal – wash and keep aside
3 cardamons
3 cloves
2 small sticks of cinnamon
2 teaspoons ginger garlic paste
1 teaspoon chillie powder
Salt to taste
3 tablespoons oil or ghee
3 tablespoons chopped coriander leaves
2 tablespoons chopped mint leaves

Heat oil/ ghee in a vessel and fry the whole spices for 2 minutes. Add the ginger garlic paste and chillie powder and sauté for a few minutes. Add the washed raw rice and dhal and stir-fry for a few minutes. Now add the coriander leaves, mint, salt and 3 cups of water and cook till the rice and dhal are soft and 'pishy-pashy'. Serve with omelet and pickle (A few pieces of chicken could also be added if desired).

---

16. Fish And Boiled Eggs Kedgeree

Serves 6   *Preparation Time 45 minutes*

Ingredients

½ kg good fleshy fish cut into thick fillets
2 cups raw rice or Basmati Rice
4 tablespoons oil
1 tablespoon ghee or butter

3 onions sliced finely

3 green chillies sliced lengthwise

4 tablespoons Moong dhal or Tur Dhal (Or any other lentils)

3 cloves

2 small sticks of cinnamon

1 teaspoon cumin powder

100 grams Sultanas or Raisins (Optional)

3 tablespoons chopped coriander leaves

2 Bay leaves

Salt to taste

1 teaspoon chillie powder

1 tablespoon lime juice / lemon juice / vinegar

6 whole peppercorns

4 hard-boiled eggs cut into quarters.

Wash the fish and cook it in a little water along with the bay leaves and salt for about 5 minutes or till the pieces are firm. Strain and keep aside. Add sufficient water to the left over fish soup to get 6 cups of liquid. Remove the bones and skin from the boiled fish and break into small pieces. Wash the Rice and dhal and keep aside.

Heat the oil in a suitable vessel and sauté the onions, cloves and cinnamon lightly. Add the slit green chillies, whole peppercorns, cumin powder and chillie powder and sauté for a few minutes. Add the rice and dhal and mix well. Now add 6 cups of the soup, limejuice / vinegar, sultanas, chopped coriander leaves and salt and cook on high heat till boiling. Reduce heat and simmer covered till the rice and dhal are cooked and slightly pasty. Gently mix in the cooked fish, butter / ghee and the hard-boiled eggs. Cover and let the rice draw in the fish for a few minutes. Serve hot or cold with Chutney or Lime Pickle.

4.

FOOGATHS AND ACCOMPANIMENTS

Foogath is the generic name for the vegetable dry side dishes served at lunch time. Vegetables such as beans, cabbage, cauliflower, greens, etc, are par boiled then tempered with mustard seeds, cumin seeds, red or green chillies, fresh grated coconut and curry leaves.

---

1. Cabbage Foogath

Serves 6   *Preparation time 30 minutes*

Ingredients

1 medium size fresh cabbage chopped finely
3 green chilies chopped
1 onion sliced
1 tablespoon chopped garlic
¼ teaspoon mustard seeds
1 sprig curry leaves
½ cup grated coconut (optional)
1 tablespoon oil
Salt to taste

Heat oil in a pan and add the mustard, garlic and curry leaves. When the mustard starts spluttering, add the chopped onion and green chilies and fry till the onions turn slightly brown. Add the Cabbage and salt and mix well. Cover and cook for about 6 to 7 minutes till the cabbage is soft. Add the grated coconut and mix well.

2. Beans Foogath

Serves 6   Preparation time 30 minutes

Ingredients

½ kg string beans chopped finely
½ cup grated coconut
3 red chilies broken into bits
¼ teaspoon mustard seeds
A few curry leaves

Boil the beans for about 5 minutes with some water. Strain and keep aside. Heat oil in a pan and add the mustard seeds. When they splutter add the red chilies and curry leaves and fry for a few seconds. Now toss in the boiled beans. Add salt and coconut and mix well. Stir-fry for a few minutes and then take down.

3. Greens Foogath

Serves 6   Preparation time 30 minutes

Ingredients

4 bunches of fresh greens
1 large onion chopped
3 green chilies chopped
Salt to taste
1 tablespoon oil
1 sprig curry leaves.
2 tablespoons grated coconut
½ teaspoon mustard seeds

Chop the greens into small bits then wash well and drain. Heat oil in a pan and add the mustard seeds. When they begin to splutter add the onions, green chillies and curry leaves and fry till the onions are slightly brown. Toss in the greens. Add salt and coconut. Cover and cook for a few minutes till all the water dries up then take down.

---

4. Beans And Carrot Foogath

Serves 6   Preparation time 30 minutes

Ingredients

½ kg string beans chopped finely
3 carrots peeled and chopped into small pieces
3 green chilies chopped
1 onion sliced
1 tablespoon chopped garlic
¼ teaspoon mustard seeds
8 curry leaves
½ cup grated coconut (optional)
1 tablespoon oil
Salt to taste

Parboil the beans and carrots in a little water for about 5 or 6 minutes. Drain and keep aside. Heat oil in a pan and add the mustard, garlic and curry leaves. When the mustard starts spluttering, add the chopped onion and green chilies and fry till the onions turn slightly brown. Add the parboiled Beans and Carrots and salt and mix well. Mix in the grated coconut. Cover and cook for a few more minutes then turn off the heat.

---

5. Snake Gourd Foogath (Serpent Gourd / Snake Coy)

Serves 6   Preparation Time 30 minutes

Ingredients

1 medium size snake gourd
3 green chilies chopped

Salt to taste
1 tablespoon oil
1 sprig curry leaves.
2 tablespoons grated coconut
½ teaspoon mustard seeds

Scrape and chop the snake gourd into small pieces then wash well and drain. Heat oil in a pan and add the mustard seeds. When they begin to splutter add the green chillies and curry leaves and fry for a few minutes. Add the snake gourd, salt and coconut. Cover and cook for a few minutes till the snake gourd is cooked and all the water dries up.

6. Radish Foogath

Serves 6   Preparation time 30 minutes

Ingredients

3 long medium size radish
3 green chilies chopped
1 onion sliced
1 tablespoon chopped garlic
¼ teaspoon mustard seeds
8 curry leaves
½ cup grated coconut (optional)
1 tablespoon oil
Salt to taste

Scrape and cut the radish into small pieces. Heat oil in a pan and add the mustard, garlic and curry leaves. When the mustard starts spluttering, add the chopped onion and green chilies and fry till the onions turn slightly brown. Add the radish and salt and mix well. Mix in the grated coconut. Cover and cook for about 5 minutes till the radish is cooked.

7. Mixed Vegetable Foogath

Serves 6   Preparation time 30 minutes

Ingredients

1 cup cauliflower florets
1 cup french beans, finely chopped
1 cup chopped carrot
½ cup green peas shelled
3 green chilies chopped
2 onions chopped
1 tablespoon chopped garlic
¼ teaspoon mustard seeds
8 curry leaves
½ cup grated coconut (optional)
1 tablespoon oil
Salt to taste

Parboil the cauliflower, beans, carrots and peas in a little water for about 5 or 6 minutes. Drain and keep aside. Heat oil in a pan and add the mustard, garlic and curry leaves. When the mustard starts spluttering add the chopped onion and green chilies and fry till the onions turn slightly brown. Add the parboiled vegetables and salt and mix well. Mix in the grated coconut. Cover and cook for about 2 more minutes then turn off the heat.

8. Green Banana Foogath

Serves 6   Preparation time 30 minutes

Ingredients

2 Raw Cooking Bananas
3 dry red chillies broken into bits
2 onions chopped
1 tablespoon chopped ginger

¼ teaspoon mustard seeds
8 curry leaves
½ teaspoon turmeric powder
½ cup grated coconut (optional)
1 tablespoon oil
Salt to taste

Peel and cut the bananas into small pieces. Heat oil in a pan and add the mustard, ginger and curry leaves. When the mustard starts spluttering, add the chopped onion and red chilies and fry till the onions turn slightly brown. Add the banana pieces, turmeric and salt and mix well. Cover and cook for a few minutes till the banana is cooked. Mix in the grated coconut.

---

9. Gherkins (Ivy Gourd) Foogath

Serves 6   *Preparation time 30 minutes*

Ingredients

300 grams tender gherkins
3 green chilies chopped
2 onions chopped
1 tablespoon chopped garlic
¼ teaspoon mustard seeds
½ teaspoon turmeric powder
8 curry leaves
½ cup grated coconut (optional)
1 tablespoon oil
Salt to taste

Cut the gherkins into thin strips. Heat oil in a pan and add the mustard, garlic and curry leaves. When the mustard starts spluttering, add the chopped onion and green chilies and fry till the onions turn slightly brown. Add the gherkins, turmeric powder and salt and mix well. Mix in the grated coconut. Cover and cook for about. 10 minutes till the gherkins are soft. Serve with rice and curry.

---

10. Dry Lady's Finger Pepper Fry (Okra Fry)

Serves 6   Preparation Time 30 minutes

Ingredients

½ kg tender lady's finger
2 teaspoons pepper powder
½ teaspoon turmeric powder
Salt to taste
2 tablespoons oil
1 teaspoon chopped garlic

Wash the whole lady's fingers and dry them well. Cut into rings discarding the ends. Mix with the pepper powder, turmeric powder, and salt. Heat oil in a pan and fry garlic and the lady's fingers till golden brown and crisp. Garnish with fried onions.

---

11. Fried Bitter Gourd

Serves 6   Preparation Time 30 minutes

Ingredients

½ kg tender bitter gourd
2 teaspoons chillie powder
½ teaspoon turmeric powder
Salt to taste
2 tablespoons oil
1 teaspoon cumin powder

Scrape and wash the bitter gourds then cut them into thin slices. Soak the slices in salt water and a pinch of turmeric for about

2 hours. Drain and squeeze out the excess water. Mix with the chillie powder, cumin powder, turmeric powder, and salt. Heat oil in a pan and fry the bitter gourd slices till golden brown and crisp.

---

12. Gherkins (Ivy Gourd) Fry

Serves 6   Preparation Time 45 minutes

Ingredients

½ kg tender gherkins
1 teaspoon chillie powder
1 teaspoon salt
1 teaspoon cumin powder
½ teaspoon turmeric powder
2 tablespoons oil

Wash the gherkins and cut them into thin slices. Mix them with the salt, chillie powder, turmeric powder and cumin powder. Heat oil in a pan and fry the gherkins till brown and crisp. Serve with rice as a side dish.

---

13. Tomato Sambal

Serves 6   Preparation Time 45 minutes

Ingredients

4 large tomatoes chopped finely
4 green chilies chopped
2 large onions sliced finely
Salt to taste
½ teaspoon pepper powder
Juice of 1 lime
2 tablespoons oil

Heat the oil in a pan and fry the onions till golden brown. Add the chopped tomatoes, chilies, salt, pepper and lime juice. Simmer on low heat till the tomatoes are cooked to a pulp and all the water dries up. Serve with rice, chapattis, etc.

---

14. Dal Mash

Serves 6   *Preparation Time 45 minutes*

Ingredients

1 cup Tur Dhal or Masur Dhal
2 onions chopped
2 green chillies chopped
1 teaspoon garlic chopped
1 teaspoon ginger chopped
½ teaspoon turmeric powder
¼ teaspoon mustard seeds
A few curry leaves
Salt to taste
1 tablespoon oil

Cook the dhal with sufficient water and ½ teaspoon turmeric powder till soft in a pressure cooker. Mash and keep aside. (The dhal should be semi solid).

Heat oil in a pan and add the mustard seeds. When it splutters add the chopped onion, green chillies curry leaves, ginger and garlic and fry well till the onions turn golden brown. Add the cooked and mashed dhal and mix well. Add a little ghee while serving.

15. Simple Dhal Curry (Dol Curry)

Serves 6   Preparation time 1 hour

Ingredients

1 cup Tur dhal or Masoor dhal
2 big tomatoes chopped
3 or 4 pods of garlic smashed
2 teaspoons chillie powder
1 teaspoon cumin powder
1 teaspoon coriander powder
½ teaspoon turmeric powder
½ teaspoon mustard seeds
2 red chilies broken into bits
A few curry leaves
1 tablespoon oil
Salt to taste

Wash the dhal and cook along with the tomatoes, turmeric, chillie powder, coriander powder, cumin powder and 3 cups of water in a pressure cooker. When the dhal is cooked, mash well, add the salt and a little more water if required.

In another vessel heat oil and add the smashed garlic, mustard, red chilies and curry leaves. When the mustard splutters pour in the cooked dhal and mix well. Serve with rice

Note: Any vegetable could be added to this Dhal Curry

16. Dhal and Greens Curry

Serves 6   Preparation Time 1 hour

Ingredients

1 cup Moong Dhal or any other dhal
1 cup of greens chopped finely . . . spinach or any other greens
2 teaspoons chillie powder
1 teaspoon coriander powder
½ teaspoon turmeric powder
2 tomatoes chopped
1 onion chopped.
Salt to taste

For the seasoning: 1 teaspoon mustard, 2 red chilies broken into bits a few curry leaves and 1 tablespoon oil.

Wash the dhal and cook it along with the greens, tomato, chillie powder, coriander powder, turmeric powder and onion with sufficient water in a pressure cooker. When done open the cooker, add salt and some more water and mash well. In another vessel, heat oil and add the mustard, broken red chilies, curry leaves and fry for some time. When the mustard starts to splutter pour in the cooked dhal. Serve with rice.

5.

ANGLO-INDIAN PICKLES AND CHUTNEYS

1. Brinjal Pickle (Aubergine / Eggplant Pickle)

Ingredients

1 kg long purple Brinjals or 1 large seedless one
3 tablespoons chillie powder
2 tablespoons chopped garlic
2 tablespoons chopped fresh ginger
1 cup vinegar
1 tablespoon mustard powder
1 tablespoon cumin powder
1 teaspoon turmeric powder
1 cup refined oil
1 cup of sugar
2 tablespoons salt

Wash and dry the Brinjals well and cut them into medium size pieces. Heat the oil in a pan. Add the ginger and garlic and sauté on low heat for a few minutes. Add the chillie powder, mustard powder, cumin powder, and turmeric powder and fry for a minute. Now add the Brinjals and salt and cook for 5 to 6 minutes on low heat. Add the vinegar and sugar and mix well. Cook till the sugar dissolves and till the brinjals are just cooked. Cool and store in bottles.

2. Mango Pickle

Ingredients

6 medium sized mangoes
3 tablespoons chillie powder
1 tablespoon fenugreek seeds ground coarsely
½ teaspoon turmeric powder
4 tablespoons salt
1 tablespoon mustard powder
1 cup Sesame oil or refined oil
½ cup vinegar
½ cup sugar

Wash and dry the mangoes well. Cut them into medium size pieces. Throw away the seeds. Mix the mango pieces with the turmeric, chillie powder, salt, fenugreek powder, mustard powder, sugar and vinegar in a stone jar and leave in the sun for a week. Shake the jar everyday so that all the mango pieces soak well. After a week, heat the oil in a pan till smoky. Cool and pour over the pickle in the jar. Mix well. The pickle is now ready for use.

3. Lime Pickle (Sweet)

Ingredients

20 medium sized limes
1 cup of sugar
3 tablespoons chillie powder
3 tablespoons salt
1 teaspoon mustard powder
½ teaspoon powdered fenugreek seeds
½ cup of vinegar
3 tablespoons oil

Cut each lime into 6 or 8 pieces, keeping 6 aside to squeeze out the juice. Steam the limes in hot water for 5 minutes till slightly soft. Dry and Cool for some time. Now mix all the ingredients, and the juice of 6 limes along with the steamed lime pieces in a pickle jar. Mix well and leave in the sun for a week. The changed appearance of the limes will show that the pickle is ready for use.

4. Hot Lime Pickle

Ingredients

20 medium sized limes
½ cup salt
1 cup sesame oil (Til Oil)
4 tablespoons chillie powder
1 tablespoon mustard powder
1 tablespoon cumin powder

Wash and dry the limes well. Cut the limes into quarters and soak with the salt in a pickle jar for a week. Shake the jar every day and leave in the sun. When the limes begin to change colour, add the chillie powder, mustard powder and cumin powder and mix well. Heat the oil in a frying pan till smoky then take down. When it cools down to room temperature, pour over the pickle and mix well. Place in the sun for a few more days.

Note: Whole slit Green chilies can also be added to this pickle if desired.

5. Fish Padda

Ingredients

500 grams sardines or small mackerels or any other small fish cut into fairly big pieces
3 tablespoons chopped garlic

2 tablespoons chopped ginger
3 tablespoons chillie powder
1 teaspoon garlic paste
1 tablespoon cumin powder
½ teaspoon turmeric powder
1 teaspoon mustard powder
2 teacups vinegar
20 or 25 curry leaves
½ lire Sesame oil or mustard oil
Salt to taste

Marinate the fish with turmeric powder & salt for half an hour. Fry the fish lightly in either sesame oil or mustard oil, for 5-8 minutes. It should only be slightly crisp. Remove & keep aside. In the same oil add the curry leaves, chopped ginger and garlic and fry for a few minutes. Mix in the garlic paste, chillie powder, cumin powder, mustard powder and salt and fry with a little vinegar till the oil seperates from the mixtures and gives out a nice aroma. Add the rest of the vinegar and the fried fish and mix well. Simmer for 2 more minutes then take down. Cool and store in bottles. This pickle will last for about 6months. Note; Instead of fresh fish, salt fish can be used instead.

6. Meat Pickle

Ingredients

½ kg boneless meat either beef or mutton cut into small bits
3 tablespoons chillie powder
½ teaspoon turmeric powder
2 teaspoons cumin powder
½ teaspoon nutmeg powder
1 teaspoon all spice powder
2 tablespoons chopped garlic
1 teaspoon chopped ginger
2 tablespoons salt
1 cup Refined Oil or Sesame oil
2 cups vinegar

Wash the meat well and leave to dry. Heat the oil in a pan and sauté the garlic and ginger for some time. Add the meat, chillie powder, cumin powder, nutmeg powder, spice powder, turmeric, vinegar and salt and mix well. Cook on low heat till the meat is cooked and the gravy is almost dry. Remove from heat and cool. When completely cold, store in Bottles and use when required (keep in the fridge).

7. Chicken Pickle

Ingredients

2 kg chicken chopped into tiny pieces
120 grams garlic
200 grams ginger
50 grams red chilies
2 tablespoons mustard powder
1 teaspoon all spice powder / garam masala powder
1 teaspoon powdered fenugreek seeds
3 cups vinegar
½ kg refined oil or Sesame oil
½ cup salt

Make a paste of the garlic, ginger, and red chilies with a little vinegar. Wash the chicken well and wipe dry. Heat oil in a vessel and fry the ground masala paste on low heat for about 3 minutes. Add the chicken pieces and mix well. Simmer for 5 minutes. Add the rest of the vinegar, salt, spice powder, mustard powder and fenugreek powder and cook on low heat till the chicken is tender and all the gravy dries up. Simmer till the oil floats on top. Cool and store in bottles. This pickle will last for a month and can be had with rice, chapattis or bread. (keep in the fridge).

8. Pork Pickle

Ingredients

½ kg boneless pork preferably without fat, cut into small bits
3 tablespoons chillie powder
½ teaspoon turmeric powder
2 teaspoons cumin powder
½ teaspoon nutmeg powder
1 teaspoon all spice powder
1 tablespoon chopped garlic
1 teaspoon chopped ginger
2 tablespoons salt
1 cup Refined Oil or Sesame oil
2 cups vinegar

Wash the pork well and leave to dry for some time. Heat the oil in a pan and sauté the garlic and ginger for some time. Add the pork, chillie powder, cumin powder, nutmeg powder, spice powder, turmeric, vinegar and salt and mix well. Cook on low heat till the meat is cooked and the gravy is almost dry. Remove from heat and cool. When completely cold, store in Bottles and use when required. (keep in the fridge).

9. Salt Fish Pickle

Ingredients

½ kg good salt fish cut into small bits
3 tablespoons chillie powder
½ teaspoon turmeric powder
1 teaspoon mustard powder
1 teaspoon cumin powder
¼ teaspoon nutmeg powder
1 tablespoon chopped ginger
1 tablespoon chopped garlic

2 tablespoons salt
1 cup Sesame oil (Til oil)
1 cup vinegar
1 teaspoon powdered fenugreek seeds

Wash the salt fish well and leave to dry for some time. Smear the turmeric powder on the Salt Fish. Heat 2 tablespoons oil in a pan and fry the Salt Fish till golden brown. Keep aside. In another pan heat the remaining oil till smoky, then turn off the heat. Add all the other ingredients and the fried salt fish and mix well. Store in bottles when cold.

10. Prawn Pickle

Ingredients

200 grams dried prawns
2 tablespoons chillie powder
½ teaspoon turmeric powder
1 tablespoon chopped garlic
2 tablespoons salt
1 teaspoon powdered mustard seeds
1 teaspoon powdered fenugreek seeds
A few curry leaves
1 cup Refined Oil
1 cup vinegar

Wash the prawns well and leave to dry in the sun for one hour. Heat 2 tablespoons oil in a pan and fry the prawns till brown. Keep aside. In another pan heat the remaining oil till smoky. Add the curry leaves and chopped garlic and fry well. Now add the chillie powder, fenugreek seeds powder, mustard powder, salt and vinegar and fry for some time. Add the prawns and mix well. Simmer for 5 minutes then remove from heat. When the pickle is cold store in bottles and use when required.

11. Prawn Balchao (A Portuguese Legacy)

Ingredients

200 grams dried prawns or shrimps
6 medium size onions chopped finely
300 grams oil
2 teaspoons chillie powder
1 tablespoon chopped garlic
1 tablespoon cumin powder
4 tablespoons vinegar

Wash the dried prawns well and remove all the sandy residue. Drain off all the water. Heat oil in a pan and fry the prawns till golden brown. Remove and keep aside. Fry the onions in the remaining oil till light brown. Add the chopped garlic, chillie powder, cumin powder and vinegar and sauté for 10 minutes. Now add the fried prawns and simmer till dry.

12. Sweet Mango Chutney Preserve

Ingredients

4 semi raw Mangoes (Poly Mangoes)
1 cup vinegar
1 cup sugar
2 tablespoons chillie powder
1 tablespoon chopped garlic
1 tablespoon chopped ginger
2 tablespoons salt
100 grams raisins
2 small sticks of cinnamon

Wash the mangoes and dry them well. Peel the skins and grate the mangoes. Discard the seeds. Add the grated mango, cinnamon and raisins to the vinegar and sugar and cook on low heat till soft. Add all the remaining ingredients and mix well.

Simmer for 5 more minutes then remove from heat. Cool and store in bottles.

---

13. Devil Chutney (Hell's Flame Chutney)

Devil Chutney is a fiery red chutney or sauce. Its bright red colour often misleads people to think that is a very pungent and spicy dish. It is actually a sweet and sour sauce and only slightly pungent. The vinegar and sugar react with the onion and red chillie to produce the bright red colour. Devil Chutney is also known as 'Hell fire or Hell's flame chutney or Fiery Mother-in-law's Tongue Chutney" due to its vivid colour.

Ingredients

2 medium size onions chopped roughly
1 teaspoon red chillie powder
1 tablespoon raisins (optional)
2 teaspoons sugar
A pinch of salt
2 tablespoons vinegar

Grind all the above ingredients together till smooth. If chutney is too thick add a little more vinegar. Serve with Coconut Rice.

---

14. Palau Chutney Or Curd Chutney

Ingredients

2 tablespoons roughly ground coconut paste
2 green chilies
2 medium size onions chopped finely
1 tablespoon chopped coriander leaves
½ teaspoon salt
1 teaspoon lime juice
½ teaspoon sugar
½ cup curds or yogurt

189

Mix all the ingredients together and serve as an accompaniment for Biryani or Palau.

---
15. Tomato Chutney

Ingredients

2 big tomatoes chopped
3 green chilies chopped
½ teaspoon cumin powder
1 tablespoon chopped garlic
1 medium size onion chopped
Salt to taste
A pinch of sugar

Heat oil in a pan and fry the onions and garlic for a few minutes. Add the chopped tomatoes, cumin powder, salt, sugar and green chilies and fry till the tomatoes are reduced to a pulp. Grind in a blender. Season with mustard seeds, red chilies and curry leaves.

---
16. Coconut Chutney

Ingredients

½ cup grated coconut
2 green chilies
½ teaspoon salt
1 tablespoon Bengal Gram / Fried Gram (this is optional and the same can be omitted)

Grind all the above to a smooth paste. Season with mustard seeds, curry leaves and a broken red chillie. This chutney is good for Dosa and Idli.

17. Coconut Chutney with Fried Salt Fish Flakes

Ingredients

2 red dry chilies
1 small onion chopped
A small ball of tamarind or ½ teaspoon tamarind paste
1 cup grated coconut
A pinch of salt
3 medium size pieces of good salt fish

Wash the salt fish well. Shallow fry the pieces in a little oil till nice and brown. Break into bits and keep aside. Grind the coconut, salt, onion, red chilies and tamarind with a little water till smooth. Add the fried bits of salt fish and mix well.

18. Mint Chutney

Ingredients

1 cup mint leaves
½ cup coriander leaves
3 green chilies
A small ball of tamarind
A small piece of ginger
1 tablespoon sugar
½ teaspoon salt

Grind all the ingredients together till smooth. This chutney can be served with rice or as a sandwich paste.

6.
SHORT CUTS AND EASIES—
Some Basic Preparations

In this section, a few basic preparations such as masala powders that can be used for every day cooking are featured. These powders can be stored for 6 to 8 months and are better than the readymade masala powders available in the shops.

1. Basic Chillie Powder

½ kg Red Chilies (long or round variety for pungency)
½ kg Kashmiri Chilies or any other variety (for adding colour)

Roast the two types of chilies in a pan for a few minutes or in a microwave oven for 1 minute. Powder them at home in the dry blender or get it done at the mill. This chillie powder can be used for any type of dish that calls for chillie powder. It can be stored for more than a year.

2. Basic Curry Powder

½ kg Red Chilies for pungency
½ kg Kashmiri Chilies or any other variety for colour
500 grams coriander seeds
200 grams cumin seeds
100 grams pepper corns
100 grams mustard seeds

Roast all the above ingredients separately then mix together and grind to a powder in a mill. A teaspoon or two of this powder can be used for almost all curries both vegetarian and non-vegetarian. It can be stored and used for more than a year.

3. Pepper Water Powder

¼ kg Red Chilies
100 grams pepper corns
100 grams cumin seeds
20 grams turmeric powder

Roast all the above ingredients separately and then grind together to a powder.

Note: 2 teaspoons of this powder should be added to 2 cups of water, 2 tomatoes chopped, a lump of tamarind and a little salt and cooked for 5 minutes to make instant pepper water. This pepper water should be seasoned with mustard, garlic and curry leaves.

4. Vindaloo Powder

½ kg red chillies
¼ kg kashmiri chillies or any other variety for colour
100 grams cumin seeds
100 grams mustard seeds
100 grams pepper corns
2 tablespoons turmeric powder

Roast all the above ingredients separately and then grind together to a powder.

Note: 2 teaspoons of this powder could be used while preparing Vindaloo using ½ kg of meat.

5. All Spice Powder (Garam Masala Powder)

2 teaspoons pepper corns
10 to 12 cloves
8 cardamoms
6 small sticks of cinnamon
1 Bay leaf
1 tablespoon fennel or saunf
1 star anise (optional)

Roast all the above lightly for a few minutes then dry grind to a fine powder. This spice powder can be used for any recipe that calls for all spice powder.

BRIDGET WHITE—ANGLO-INDIAN RECIPE BOOKS

1 **A COLLECTION OF ANGLO-INDIAN ROASTS, CASSEROLES AND BAKES** is a practical and easy guide to the preparation of a variety of Anglo-Indian Roasts, Casseroles and Bakes such as Shepherd's Pie, Washer-man's Pie, Roast Chicken, Roast Turkey, etc.

2. **ANGLO-INDIAN DELICACIES** is a collection of Recipes of popular vintage and contemporary Cuisine of Colonial India such as Pork Bhooni, Devil Pork Curry, Calcutta Cutlets, Fish Kedegeree, Double Onions Meat Curry, Camp Soup, Bengal Lancers Shrimp Curry, etc.

3. **THE ANGLO-INDIAN FESTIVE HAMPER** is a collection of popular Anglo-Indian Festive and Holiday Treats, such as Cakes, Sweets, Christmas goodies, Puddings, Sandwiches, Preserves, Home-made Wines, etc,

4. **THE ANGLO-INDIAN SNACK BOX** is a collection of simple and easy to follow recipes of tasty `snacks, short eats, nibbles and finger food, which includes savouries, sandwiches, wraps, rolls, pastries, sweets etc

5. **VEGETARIAN DELICACIES** is a collection of simple and easy recipes of delectable Vegetarian Dishes. The repertoire is rich and vast, ranging from simple Soups and Salads, to mouth watering Curries, Stir fries, Rice dishes, Casseroles, Baked Dishes and popular Accompaniments. The book also highlights the health benefits and the goodness of each vegetable.

ALSO BY BRIDGET WHITE- A NOSTALGIC BOOK ON KGF

"Kolar Gold Fields—Down Memory Lane" undertakes a nostalgic journey of almost 150 years, beginning with the historical and mythological origins of the Kolar Gold Mines, its golden progress through the years under the John Taylor and Sons Company, its gradual decline, and the final closure of the once prosperous Kolar Gold Mining Company in 2003. Thus ending a golden chapter in History, which now lies buried in the annals of time.

It recalls the glorious and cosmopolitan life led by the tiny vibrant Anglo-Indian Community (a living legacy of the British Raj) in the early days of KGF who lived in sprawling bungalows with beautiful gardens and domestic helpers at their beck and call. It recalls the grand Christmas Balls and Dances held at the Skating Rink and the Jam Sessions and Pound Parties in Buffalo Lodge.

It finally focuses on the author's childhood memories of growing up in KGF in the 1950s and 60s, and of life's many simple pleasures—home, family, school, playmates, entertainments, games, etc. It recalls memories of old familiar haunts and landmarks of KGF and the people who were an indispensable part of life in those days. The book succeeds in capturing and preserving the ethos and naunces of a bygone era.

http://memoriesofkgf.blogspot.com

ABOUT THE AUTHOR
BRIDGET WHITE-KUMAR

Bridget White-Kumar
Cookery book Author, Food Consultant and Culinary Historian

Bridget White-Kumar is a Cookery Book Author, Food Consultant and Culinary Historian. She has authored 7 Recipe books on Anglo-Indian Cuisine. Her area of expertise is in Colonial Anglo-Indian Food and she has gone through a lot of effort in reviving the old forgotten dishes of the Colonial British Raj Era. Her 7 Recipe books are a means of preserving for posterity, the very authentic tastes and flavours of Colonial 'Anglo' India, besides recording for future generations, the unique heritage of the pioneers of Anglo-Indian Cuisine.

Her Recipe book *ANGLO-INDIAN CUISINE—A LEGACY OF FLAVOURS FROM THE PAST* that was published in India, was recently selected as *'Winner from India'* by *GOURMAND INTERNATIONAL SPAIN,* Under the Category: *'BEST CULINARY HISTORY BOOK'.* This prestigious Award is 'THE OSCARS' for Cook book writers. Awards are given every year for various categories and genres ie for Cook Book Authors, Cook Books, Chefs, Wine makers, etc. who compete from all over the world.

Bridget is also an **Independent Freelance Consultant on Food Related matters.** She has assisted many Restaurants, Hotels and Clubs in Bangalore and elsewhere with her knowledge of Colonial Anglo-Indian Food besides helping them to revamp and reinvent their Menus by introducing new dishes which are a combination of both Continental and Anglo-Indian. Many of them are now following the Recipes and guidance given by her and the dishes are enjoyed by both Indian and Foreign Guests.

Bridget also conducts Cooking Demonstrations and Workshops at various places across the country such as Clubs, Restaurants, Women's Groups, Corporate Offices, etc. She is always ready to share and talk about Recipes and Food.

She can be contacted on **+919845571254**

Email bridgetkumar@yahoo.com
http://bridgetkumar.wordpress.com
http://anglo-indianfood.blogspot.com
http://anglo-indianrecipes.blogspot.com
http://bridgetrecipes.blogspot.com

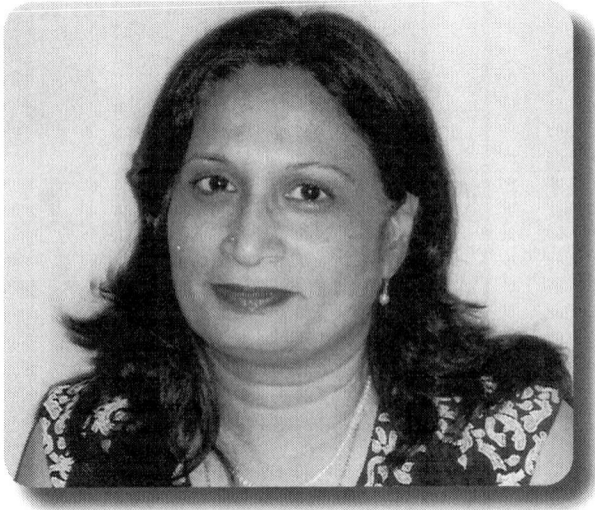

37696978R00132

Printed in Great Britain
by Amazon